More Advance Praise for *Crooked Smile:*

"I have really struggled to confine my enthusiasm to so few words. First, this is a story that will bring hope to so many families who live the horror that the Cohens experienced as a result of Daniel's injury. More importantly, it is a book for a much broader audience, because it is so well written. Lainie has the artistic talent to transport the reader and make one a part of the family. From the pastoral opening scenes at the lake through all the pain and anxiety through to the triumphs, one is emotionally drawn into the story in quite an extraordinary way.

Each year in Canada, at least 4,000 families will experience the shock of learning that a loved one has suffered a brain injury. They will live the agony of waiting for news; the frustration of not knowing the outcome, and the exhaustion of seemingly endless hospital visits. Few, if any, will have a Lainie Cohen who can invite the reader to be a part of the family as she chronicles the journey that is an on-going part of her son Daniel's recovery from brain injury; a journey that speaks profoundly of the power of love and determination as a valuable adjunct to medical science."

— John Kumpf, Executive Director,
Ontario Brain Injury Association

"This book brings back memories of what we, as a family, went through under similar circumstances and learned that no matter what, *never give up.*"

— Parnelli Jones, winner of the Indianapolis 500

Crooked Smile

Published by ECW PRESS
2120 Queen Street East, Suite 200, Toronto, Ontario, Canada M4E 1E2

NATIONAL LIBRARY OF CANADA CATALOGUING IN PUBLICATION DATA

Cohen, Lainie
Crooked smile : one family's journey toward healing / Lainie Cohen.

ISBN 1-55022-573-1

1. Cohen, Lainie — Family. 2. Sick children — Family relationships.
3. Adjustment (Psychology) 4. Caregivers — Canada — Biography. 1. Title.

RC387.5.C636 2003   155.9'16   C2002-905421-4

Editor: Jennifer Hale
Cover and Text Design: Tania Craan
Production & Typesetting: Mary Bowness
Printing: Transcontinental

This book is set in AGaramond and John Handy

The publication of *Crooked Smile* has been generously supported by the Canada Council, the Ontario Arts Council, and the Government of Canada through the Book Publishing Industry Development Program. **Canadä**

DISTRIBUTION
CANADA: Jaguar Book Group, 100 Armstrong Avenue, Georgetown, ON, L7G 5S4

PRINTED AND BOUND IN CANADA

ECW PRESS
ecwpress.com

Crooked Smile

ONE FAMILY'S JOURNEY TOWARD HEALING

For Westwind,
Remember to facilitate hope.
Lainie Cohen

LAINIE COHEN

ECW PRESS

Acknowledgements

My family and I have been blessed by many gifts from many givers. To all of you, too numerous to list here, who have crossed our paths on our journey toward healing, I'd like to express our heartfelt gratitude. I'd also like to thank those who helped move this story from an exercise in healing to reality.

Thanks to Ann Ireland, writer-in-residence at the Toronto Reference Library, who read an excerpt from the first draft and encouraged me to continue.

I'd like to acknowledge the significant contribution of Lesley Krueger — teacher, editor, and mentor — whose insightful comments taught me to go deeper to get to the heart of the story.

The feedback from my Ryerson classmates was invaluable. Thanks to past and present writing group members: Diana Armstrong, Paul Babiak, Pauline Berenik, Cathy Buchanan, Steve Cline, Brian Francis, Jay Millar, Kate Moore, Mike Ongarato, and Noni Regan. Special thanks to Noni for copy editing.

Thanks to writers Jon Weiner and Deborah Heiligman and poets Merle Nudelman and Jacqueline Borowick for their generous advice and support. And special mention to my son-in-law Scott Friedmann for his involvement as first reader and personal booster.

I am grateful to Dr. Peter Rumney for reviewing the medical data and terminology. I assume full responsibility for any errors or omissions.

Thanks to Jack David and Jen Hale of ECW Press for recognizing the potential of this work. Jen's cheerful guidance and Jack's reasonableness ensured that all obstacles were overcome. It's been a pleasure working with them and their staff.

I am deeply indebted to my children: Alyssa, Daniel, and Jonathan, and my husband, Joel, who allowed me to share their story with honesty and candour. It is with their loving support that I offer this story, hoping it will benefit others.

Most of all, I wish to thank my husband Joel, my partner on this journey. His love and incredible determination have no bounds.

For my mother

Leona Mensch Garmaise

1919–2002

Part One

CHAPTER ONE

When I awake, the cottage is hushed. The kids are still sleeping, but Joel is already on the screened-in porch, eating breakfast and reading a section from yesterday's newspaper. No need to hurry here, a place where time doesn't matter. That's one of the things I love about it. That and the calm glassy lake that beckons my canoe. I grab a plum and brush Joel's bent neck with my lips before setting off across the bay.

Little things are etched into my memory of that Sunday, the last one of August, such as Jonathan parading around with the canoe overhead. "Mom, this is how I portaged on our trips in the wilderness. Remember, it was much harder with all those mosquitoes and a seventy-pound pack on my back."

I marvel at the lean muscles in his fourteen-year-old arms. My youngest child looks so much like his father, the same lanky build, gangling legs, long skinny face. He and Joel share the same colouring too, fair skinned with green-grey eyes, just like Alyssa, our eldest. Right now, she's relaxing in the hammock, enjoying some light summer reading before boring into her university texts. She stretches. Her skimpy bikini straps pull tautly and then settle back into place. Even when she crosses her ankles, her thighs don't touch.

Maybe in my next life, I'll look like that: five-foot-four, slim, and with cleavage. I stare down at my thighs, rubbing together on the edge of the dock. Middle-aged spread indeed. At least no varicose veins spider their way up my legs yet. I unbutton my beach top and slip into the water, swimming a few laps of front crawl back and forth between my neighbour's dock and ours. As I dry off, Daniel and his friends stride down to the lake, flicking each other with their towels. Three of his friends are spending the weekend, so we've had a full house of laughter, music, and the constant roar of the boat engine. Water-skis, kneeboards, tubes — it doesn't matter. The boys are happy to be pulled on anything so long as they can go fast.

"Hi, guys. Had any breakfast?"

"Yes. Thanks for the blueberry muffins, Mrs. Cohen," John says. "They were delicious."

Daniel doesn't waste any words. Peeling off his T-shirt and exposing a bronzed tan, he dives off the end of the dock, barely rippling the surface; his powerful arms slice through the water. When he emerges from the lake, he shakes his head back and forth like our dog, squeezes the excess water from his long hair, and then pulls it back into a ponytail. He'll never have to worry about being bald like his father, I think. Daniel has my family's thick dark hair, deep brown eyes, and long eyelashes that his sister so envies. I turn to look at my husband, whose shiny dome is covered by a wide brimmed hat, even in the shade. No point taking any chances, he feels. Grey hairs sneak out from behind his ears and infiltrate his trim brown beard.

Was it just last month that we celebrated our twenty-fifth anniversary? Our first holiday in years without the children — what a treat! Ten days of touring the Normandy coast through towns of cobble-stoned streets and stone houses so close to the road that I could practically pick the flowers from the window-boxes as we drove by. I recall the fragrance of fresh ocean air and the smell of buttery croissants wafting from the patisseries. I look at Joel absorbed in his book and think about walking hand-in-hand through paths in the woods, my head just brushing his shoulder.

"Hey, Dad. We're low on gas. Where's your credit card?"

Daniel bounds up to the cottage and quickly returns, swinging the boat key in one hand. The credit card is tucked into the waistband of his bathing suit. He and his friends scramble into the boat. The dog jumps in too, claiming her favourite seat on the right-hand side of the boat just behind the driver. When he pats her, she settles down, curling up with her head neatly resting on her paws.

He primes the engine. It revs briefly, then sputters and dies. "Dad, when are you going to replace this tub with a real ski boat?"

"Maybe when you give up camp, so you can use it. It serves us just fine," Joel replies.

The engine roars to life again, drowning any further talk. Daniel reverses the boat slowly out of the boat port. When the bow is pointing eastward, he guns the motor and takes off down the bay.

After lunch, Alyssa announces, "I'd like to leave soon so I don't have to sit in traffic for hours. Besides, I've made plans tonight. Daniel, do you want to drive back with me?"

"Naw, I'll catch a ride later with one of the guys. They're talking about heading out to another cottage soon, but one of them will be driving back around five."

Joel and I welcome the quiet that descends when our son and his friends leave. My husband pours himself a glass of red wine and I arrange a plate of veggies and dip to nibble on. We walk back to the dock together, finding the bay peaceful now with the boaters gone. The other shoreline is already in shadow, the sharpness and rough edges of the pine and spruce needles transformed into blurry smudges of green. Silver slivers of birch reflect in the stillness of the water. In the quiet, there's just the sound of our voices and the swish of a canoe paddle. The lengthening shadows signal us. Reluctantly, we gather our things and head back to the cottage. During dinner, we watch as the sun — burnishing to a coppery ball — begins its slow descent behind the hillside.

Jonathan is setting up the video he's rented when the phone rings.

"I'll get it," he shouts and seconds later calls out, "Mom and Dad, take the phone. It's Alyssa."

I pick up the phone in the kitchen and Joel gets on the extension in our bedroom.

"Hi, Alyss," I say cheerily. "I thought you were going out

tonight."

Her voice trembles and cracks in reply, "It's about Daniel." She relays the message in telegraphic fragments: "Police called . . . car crash . . . both boys thrown . . . no seatbelts on . . ."

"What? Where is he?"

"York County Hospital."

"Is he okay?" Joel asks.

"Badly hurt. Head injury — that's all they said. John was hurt too. Got to go. Meet me there."

I don't remember starting to scream, but a wail reverberates throughout the house. Jonathan comes running into the kitchen to find me clutching at Joel for support. The phone receiver dangles down the kitchen wall, swinging like a coiled serpent.

"What's wrong?" he cries.

In a voice that's lost its usual control, Joel blurts, "Daniel's been hurt. We've got to go."

Like robots, my husband and I start to go through the motions of closing windows and locking doors. Jonathan stands there, dazed, uncertain what to do.

"Go to the Gordons'," Joel says.

Jonathan races next door. As I'm tying up my sneakers, he rushes back in with our neighbour, Marilyn.

"Don't worry. I'll manage," Marilyn says.

She hugs me before we hurry off.

It feels cold in the car and I move the air vent, deflecting it into the back where my youngest sits silently. The winding road from our cottage is only three kilometres long and when we reach the highway, Joel picks up speed. Traffic is moving well here. He reaches for my hand and grips it on top of the stick shift. The knob feels solid in my palm and his fingers warm mine.

We are cut off from life in our enclosed space. Joel and I ask each other questions that neither can answer. What has happened? Will Daniel be okay? All our hopes rest on news from the cellphone that doesn't ring.

We pass familiar sights: two marinas, the garden centre, a video store, and the stand selling wild blueberries with its Sold Out sign in place. Fields of empty corn stalks form darkening shadows at the side of the road. Now and then neon lights flicker from a roadside doughnut shop or gas station.

Joel phones the hospital and speaks briefly to a staff member in Emergency.

"Your son is unconscious and has just been transferred to the trauma unit at Sunnybrook Hospital."

"Does our daughter know?"

"We tried to call her but there's no answer at your home. She's probably en route here."

Joel hangs up and immediately dials his brother's number. "David, I need you to go to Sunnybrook Hospital." He relays the little information we know. "If you hear any news at all, please call us."

I'm startled to see Joel smashing his hand against the dashboard. "That goddamn kid. Has he no brains? Why wasn't he wearing a seatbelt? I bet they were going too fast. Daniel always drove too quickly. I told him, but did he listen? No! Remember when he took the turn too quickly and went into a ditch? Smashed up the car. Wish he had hurt himself then."

"What? You wanted him to be hurt?"

"Not a lot. Just a little. So he would've learned a lesson."

"Joel, Daniel wasn't even driving today. It was his friend, John, remember?" I touch his hand and he returns it to the stick shift. My fingers cover his.

"I know." He glances briefly at me, his face contorting with pain. "Did you see that car John was driving? A small car. I hate small cars for teenage drivers. I should never have let him go in it. Should have insisted he go home with Alyssa."

"That's crazy. He came up with John. He wanted to go back with him."

"I shouldn't have let him."

This isn't our fault, I want to say. Then I question myself. Did we do something wrong? I think back to all those years I spent driving carpool to hockey practices and games. A mother whose head couldn't even be seen from behind the headrest of the largest station wagon on the market. Thump. A hockey bag thrown in the back. The slam of the door and then the click. The sound of the seatbelt fastening. Three boys, three clicks. Daniel knew I was a stickler for the rules. My car didn't move unless all the seatbelts were on. What went wrong?

The landscape passes in a blur of darkness, familiar shapes transformed into the menacing unknown.

We're racing. I glance at the speedometer and yell at Joel, "Are you nuts? Slow down! There's already one of us in the hospital."

The car slows and we drift back into silence. I start to shiver despite the summer's heat and place my hands under my bottom to warm them. The leather seat feels so cold. I gaze forward, mesmerized by the trail of red lights ahead, two abreast, then three when the highway widens. We're still an hour's drive away from the city.

I think of hospital emergency rooms — the bright lights, sticky vinyl chairs, and long waits. Like many parents with active kids, we've had our time there, anxiously anticipating the results of X-rays and then waiting patiently for the fitting of splints, plastering of casts, or sizing of crutches. Only once, when we raced to the hospital with Jonathan in the midst of an asthma attack, did I feel as much panic as I do now.

Another twenty minutes pass and still there's no call from Alyssa or David. Joel phones Sunnybrook's emergency room. Over the speakerphone I hear a female voice, "A doctor is with your son. We'll call you back when the doctor is done."

"Please, tell me," I ask, "is he alive?"

The nurse avoids answering by simply repeating her previous message. Joel presses the end button as I start to keen, "We've lost him."

Jonathan leans forward from the back seat and holds my shoulders firmly while I wail; his father clenches the steering wheel and curses the traffic that has slowed almost to a standstill. My chest continues to heave as my sobs subside.

If the doctor is still with him, then Daniel must be alive, we reason. Beneath this hope lurks the worry that Alyssa and David would not share news of his death over a cellphone.

Joel turns on the radio. The reporter announces, "Traffic is unusually heavy on Highway 400 due to heavy volume and construction delays. The alternate routes are also very busy. Stay tuned for an update in fifteen minutes. This report is brought to you by . . ."

At long last, we reach the emergency department. A nurse immediately ushers us into a small waiting room. In the cramped space are Alyssa, David and his wife Roz, my brother Yaron and his wife Sue, and two of our friends. How did they know to come? We grab Alyssa and clasp her to us. Her body quakes as she nods tearfully, "He's alive."

Then we notice the stranger — a young doctor with the traditional white coat. How could I not see him standing there?

"Your son has a massive blood clot in his brain. He's being operated on right now." The doctor tips his head towards Alyssa. "Your daughter, here, signed the permission papers. Why don't you all wait upstairs? You'll be more comfortable there. The procedure should take about two hours."

We're led to an elevator and invited to wait in the visitor's lounge on the seventh floor near the surgical intensive care unit. The room is filled with couches and chairs, a room that could be considered comfortable in other circumstances. But we find no comfort here. The room is empty, save for us, and the silence eerie. The only sounds heard are the ones we make. No hustle and bustle of emergency room clamour. No P.A. system announcing calls for physicians. There's a hushed solemnity in the room and our friend Al's voice seems to boom with its forced cheeriness.

"Daniel is strong. He'll be okay. You'll see."

We want to believe him.

David drapes his arm around Joel and together they pace back and forth around the room. When I collapse on a couch, Yaron and Alyssa hug me. The others stand around, trying to offer support to Jonathan, who looks frozen in place like a deer startled by car headlights. Which way can he bolt?

Someone boils the kettle and makes cups of tea. I hold the cup without drinking, warming my fingers on the porcelain. Pressing the cup against my belly, I wait.

The door to the lounge opens and we jump up anxiously. The chaplain, in a dark suit suggestive of mourning, walks in and introduces himself. He sits and talks but I don't hear his words. I watch his fingers splayed out against his knees. His right arm lifts gracefully as he gestures his concern like a conductor in front of an orchestra. Sinking against the plush cushions of the couch, I sip my tea. Consolation seems far away.

Shortly after the chaplain leaves, the door opens again and a large woman in a white uniform enters. Her face is broad and serious-looking but her voice is caring, "How are you coping?"

"My stomach is churning," I reply. "I've been to the washroom five times already."

"I'm sorry I can't dispense any medication to you directly. Why don't you go to the emergency room to get something? Don't worry. You have time. We won't hear from the surgeon for at least an hour yet."

My friend, Ellen, comes with me back downstairs. It's strange approaching the emergency room from inside the hospital. Everything seems backwards, as if we were rewinding a video and watching the jerky actions unfold in reverse. This time, as we wait in the usual place, my back rubs impatiently against a vinyl chair. I feel foolish to be here — in an emergency room for an upset stomach — and I'm worried that there will be a long delay, but I'm seen quickly and receive some pills.

Ellen and I head outdoors. The night air is crisp and stars light the dark sky, each one shining in place, unaware of any earthly crisis. We decide to take a short walk and pass by K-Wing, the veterans' nursing home section of the hospital. My seventy-nine-year-old father lives there. I visit him often and think about the quality of his life. My father's former erect walk has turned into a shuffle as he peers into rooms looking for his mother. "Have you seen her today? She knit this sweater for me. I wanted to thank her and ask her to take me home."

Life is not like literature. We cannot make deals offering to trade our earthly goods, or to barter one's life for another, although for a fleeting moment that thought crosses my mind.

I think about death — my father-in-law's fatal heart attack in mid-July. It was so unexpected, but he was seventy-five; our son is only seventeen-and-a-half. My thoughts race with fear. Joel and I recognized Daniel's immaturity and saw him struggling to establish an identity. He so often wanted to do things his way and was prepared to take foolish chances. How could he and his friend have been in such a hurry that they would take such risks? With all the training he's had and with our constant reminders, how could he ride in a car without wearing a seatbelt? I'm so angry with him for almost destroying himself.

At 1:30 a.m. the neurosurgeon strides into the visitor's lounge. Her green cap is slightly askew, allowing brown curls to escape onto her forehead. She shows no signs of fatigue despite the late hour, exuding an air of confidence and accomplishment. Alyssa, Joel, Jonathan, and I cling to one another. Gathering around, our friends and family create a circle of palpable support.

The surgeon is frank with us. "I've just removed a massive blood clot that was fairly deep in Daniel's brain. Had this happened to an older person, I wouldn't even have tried to operate, but he has age and strength in his favour. The first seventy-two hours are critical. His chances of survival are about eighty per cent."

She tempers the positive by warning us of the dangers: possible seizures, internal haemorrhaging, or build-up of intracranial pressure.

"I've left a flap open in his skull to accommodate brain swelling, and I'm prepared to operate again if necessary," she tells us. "Because of the location of the blood clot, I expect that there'll be residual neurological damage, probably affecting expressive speech and motor areas on Daniel's right side. The other doctors will close up and finish the operation. It will be several hours before you may see him."

As the doctor leaves, I look around the room. Everyone looks drained. Joel's shoulders are sagging and Jonathan can barely stand upright. My whole body feels numb, as if I've just had a giant injection of freezing to prevent the awareness of pain. My mind seems frozen too. Words bounce into resistant barriers and refuse to form coherent thoughts. Inside my bubble, I hear Joel's voice take charge.

"There's no point in all of us being here. Alyssa can take Jonathan home. Lainie and I will wait to see Daniel."

Jonathan looks relieved, as if hearing his father's voice — once more in control — guarantees that everything will turn out all right.

"I'm staying too," Alyssa says.

"We'll take Jonathan home with us," David and Roz offer.

When everyone leaves, we continue our vigil.

At 4:45 a.m. Joel, Alyssa, and I are finally allowed into the surgical intensive care unit to see Daniel. As we walk down the hall, Joel pulls ahead, his stride like that of a speed walker approaching the end of a race, determined and fatigued. Alyssa and I clasp hands. We pass white-curtained windows before we approach his bed. I can see the steady rise and fall of his chest under the crisp sheet. My heart races. My son is alive!

His eyes are closed and his face looks so still. Cheeks and chin, darkened with shadow, are almost hidden behind the pale blue tube that snakes from his mouth to the ventilator on the wall, controlling his breathing. His head is wrapped in white gauze bandages covered by a blue cap; the indigo corona pierced by a thin wire poking out above his left eyebrow. My gaze follows the wire to a machine that flashes with bright shiny lines and buzzes in a language I don't understand.

Joel and I are stricken dumb as we stand by our son's side. But Alyssa reaches out and touches him gently on his right arm that rests at his side.

"Daniel, we're here now. You're fine. Everything is going to be fine."

My voice croaks as my throat tries to squeeze out words: "Daniel, we love you."

All Joel can manage is, "Daniel."

Our legs are rubbery when we turn to leave. We walk as if our feet were bound together, Joel in the middle, his arms weighted on our shoulders. Somehow we make our way back to the car. Alyssa drives home.

CHAPTER TWO

It's early January and snowing outside. It's been over five years now since Daniel's injury and I sit, staring out the patio doors of my kitchen to the backyard that stretches as long as an empty football field. Everything is blanketed in white. Heavy powder covers the picnic table like thick icing applied by an absent-minded baker. Drifts of windswept snow fill in the open slats of the wooden deck and pile high against the frosted glass door. An icy wind howls from the north. I turn on the radio.

"It's 9:00 a.m. Here's a brief weather update before the news," the announcer says. "We're expecting more snow in Toronto today. Motorists are advised to leave their cars at home and take public transportation."

I turn off the radio. I hadn't planned to go anywhere today so I didn't mind when Joel took my car, the one with a four-wheel drive, to work.

It's a good day to start writing my book, I tell myself. I've wanted to do this for a while, to write Daniel's story for him. I'd like to try to recapture events to help him understand that period of time for which he has no memory.

When I leave the kitchen, the puppy starts to whine. She scratches the wooden gate secured across the doorway. I hadn't realized she would be so needy. Every time I take a step, she follows me and tries to nestle on my toes. She whimpers until I'm back in sight. I set up my laptop computer on the kitchen table and plug it in. The puppy cuddles contentedly on my feet. As a young girl, I always preferred to do my homework in the warmth of the kitchen rather than in my own room. Perhaps this new venue will spur my writing along. The task seems daunting.

Life has turned out to be different than anything I might have imagined on that late August day and I'm not sure where to begin. Our lives seemed so settled then. I was working full-time as a psychoeducational consultant for the York Region school board and Joel was a senior partner at Richter, a chartered accountancy firm. Just the month before, we had celebrated our twenty-fifth wedding anniversary with a tour of the Normandy coast and the Loire Valley in France. It was such a golden time in our lives and we laughingly recalled the importance of fate, how we were fixed up on a blind date when we were both undergraduate students in Montreal, our hometown. We talked a lot on that holiday, reminiscing about the plans we'd made for our lives and the successes and surprises we experienced.

In 1970, we moved to Toronto for Joel to get his MBA. To support us, I took a job teaching grades two and three in a private school. Joel never completed that degree. Instead he took a summer job with Richter that turned into his life's work. I continued teaching while raising our family. After five years of marriage, we had the first of our three children, spaced about three years apart. When our youngest child entered grade one, I started graduate studies in psychology and special education, later becoming a consultant, specializing in the assessment of children.

I think back to that last innocent summer. Our daughter Alyssa was working in Joel's office doing an internship in accounting. Aged twenty, she had completed the first two years of a four-year degree program in social sciences at the University of Western Ontario and had just been accepted into the school's prestigious honours business administration program. She planned to become an accountant like her dad. In high school, she had shown an entrepreneurial bent — organizing swim lessons at the cottage, tutoring students in math and French, and compiling practice tests in other subjects that she sold to students anxious to improve their grades. And she was such a social being. She seemed to live with one ear attached to a phone receiver, constantly talking to her boyfriend or one of her many girlfriends.

Daniel was different. He was so much quieter, at least at home. He, too, was a social creature, but he guarded his relationships and seldom spoke to us about his friends. Nor did he show the same interest in academic achievement as his sister. Where she strived for perfection, he followed the school of "it's good enough," content with Cs and Bs, although he was certainly capable of higher grades. If he hadn't dropped calculus, he would have completed his high school studies in June, at age seventeen and a half. As it was, he was planning to return for one more semester, but he had no specific career direction. He talked of going to university in British Columbia the following year, so he could be close to the ski hills. He joked about becoming a ski bum. We knew he hoped to get a job at Whistler, B.C., when he finished his semester in January. His energy was always focussed on sports activities. That's where he shone, and he managed to make it look effortless.

Some days I wondered if he would end up as a physical education teacher, or perhaps a sports psychologist. He really liked kids, and enjoyed working with them at camp as a water-ski instructor. He had also taught swimming, but preferred his part-time job in a restaurant where he could work longer hours, earning more money to maintain the used car we had bought him.

Jonathan, only fourteen, wanted so much to be like his older brother. He had even started to grow his hair long, so he could have a ponytail too. In winter, Jonathan played competitive hockey, although playing defence and not forward meant he didn't score as many goals as Daniel did. In summer, he went to the same camp where Daniel, as part of the ski staff, was treated with such respect. But Jonathan showed no interest in water-skiing.

"If you don't want water-skiing, then you'd better become a tripper," Daniel advised. "Being a regular counsellor sucks."

So Jonathan reluctantly went out on a canoe trip and found to his surprise that he liked it. After that, he signed up for another trip. And then another. Jonathan was like that. Slow to get started and then — wham. By the end of the summer, he had won the award for the most trip days of any camper.

At school he had shown the same pattern. In his early elementary years, Jonathan had some difficulty learning to read and write, but when he completed grade eight he was one of the top three students in his school. And popular too. Just like his older brother and sister.

Things were almost too good to be true. I remember feeling grateful and cherishing each moment of those golden days Joel and I spent in France. There was no reason then to expect that our lives would be different from what we imagined. We would eventually live and travel as empty nesters, our children grown and self-sufficient, coming back to visit with noisy grandchildren. The future looked bright indeed.

Then came August 29.

CHAPTER THREE

Can time disappear into a vacuum? Monday and Tuesday engulf us. We have little sense of minutes or hours passing in the hospital visitor's lounge. I feel numb, disconnected from anyone else around me, except Joel, whose hand I hold. We want to spend all our time with our son, but we're allowed to see him for only five or ten minutes per hour. His schedule must accommodate doctors' rounds, physiotherapist's activities, and numerous tests and procedures.

Every time we walk down the hall to the surgical intensive care unit, we picture Daniel sitting up, eager to talk, and reassuring us that all will be fine. Instead, we're faced with a waxlike figure lying inert in bed. His face and body look whole. He's broken no bones and has few scratches or abrasions except around his right elbow.

But a cotton cap covers his head, hiding the operation's scars and his missing ponytail. And machines surround him, beeping and buzzing as his vital signs and functions are monitored and controlled. Deep in a coma, can he hear us calling his name? Can he feel my touch on his cheek? So soft now, not stubbly in his usual manner with three days of scruffy growth.

Where is my son? Amidst the bright lights, he is lost in darkness.

We feel lost too. Our legs wobble as we walk away from his bedside, linked arms supporting each other. The elevator makes stops on several floors. When other passengers enter, I bury my tear-stained face against Joel's shoulder.

In the privacy of our car, Joel slams his hand against the steering wheel. "Why did this happen? How could he be so stupid? He's thrown his life away."

"Don't say that. The doctor says he'll still have a good life."

"Really? What kind of life will that be?"

"Nobody knows." I place my hand on his arm. "We just have to hope."

"I hate this waiting . . . not knowing." His voice softens to a whimper as he wipes tears away with the back of his hand, brushing mine away. I pull my hand back and, wrapping my arms around my shoulders, try to comfort myself.

On Wednesday morning, Joel is still sleeping, so I leave for the hospital on my own. When I arrive a little after 9:00 a.m., the elevator is not working. I trudge up the seven flights of stairs to the visitor's lounge. Puffing and red-faced, I approach the volunteer at the reception desk. Above the pink smock is a head of soft grey curls and a warm smile.

"Daniel Cohen, please," I say, trying to catch my breath. She picks up the phone and calls the surgical intensive care unit.

"I'm sorry, you'll have to wait. He's having physiotherapy now. They'll call back when he's done."

I borrow a pen and some paper and start to write down my thoughts. Will Daniel ever regain consciousness? What will he be like? How many movies have we watched that feature themes of disabilities, diseases, and disfigurement? Will he be strong? Fight to live? Will we help him or be in his way? How will we cope with the pressure, the uncertainty, the waiting?

Constant waiting for very small changes to occur. Hiding sorrow and tears and smiling. Saying false words of hope; words we want to believe in. Painting pictures of what was — healthy, active, athletic: racing down a ski hill on the edge of control, slaloming on water skis so proud of the speed, jumping and making the basketball shot, playing hockey with his friends, then coming in all sweaty and offering to give me a hug. This was my son.

I keep thinking about him, wondering whether I can find any clues in his personality or behaviour to make sense of this unfathomable event. In so many ways he seemed a typical teenager with a pendulum swing of emotions and goals. He spent most of his time with his friends and not us, but we expected that and hoped for a healthy separation.

Daniel defined himself by his athletic prowess, not by his academic pursuits, but he had visions of university, of moving on in life, even though his goals were unclear. He prided himself on his mellowness, a "laid-back attitude" that we sometimes felt was a cover for rumbling uncertainty beneath. He showed little patience for reading unless the book was action-packed and fast moving, yet he could watch TV for hours. He mastered video games readily and could beat all his friends in his favourite hockey game.

Sometimes when I'd come home from work, I'd have to wend my way through a pile of knapsacks and smelly sneakers. Daniel and one friend would be on the floor in front of the TV, while the other guys sprawled on the couch behind them drinking soft drinks and eating chips. He always looked so intent as he manoeuvred the control to knock out his opponents on the screen.

"Shit! Not another goal," his friend would groan.

"Better luck next time," he replied. "Anyone else want to take me on?"

At other times, he showed a warmth and sensitivity beyond his years. When he was a first-year counsellor at camp, a troubled fourteen-year-old camper confided in him, knowing that Daniel would listen and care. Recognizing that he couldn't resolve the boy's severe homesickness on his own, he shared his concerns with the camp director. Then he spent extra time with the camper until the boy's father could pick him up from camp.

I think of the many visits he made to his grandfather in the nursing home, never challenging his grandfather's confused ramblings even when their conversation resembled a play from the Theatre of the Absurd, with no meaningful exchanges at all.

Most of all he had the spirit of a little boy who wanted to play, within the body of a young man. Now I pray he has the chance to grow up and become that man I dreamed he would be.

Thursday, 3:00 a.m. and I'm not sleeping. Fluffing my pillow, I pull on an extra blanket and try to relax. Fifteen minutes later, I opt to take half a sleeping pill and lie down in bed to try again. At 4:00 a.m., still unsuccessful, I head down to the kitchen for some hot chocolate. While waiting for the kettle to boil, I call the hospital and speak to Mike, the night nurse.

"Daniel opened his eyes several times during the night, but they aren't focussed. He's still unconscious. We're hoping to wean him from the respirator today and have him breathing on his own."

I sigh with relief, as there appears to be some sign of progress. I'm grateful that the nurses and doctors are so supportive. They try to answer every question, but are unable to make predictions or give us the time-lines that we so desperately want. Everyone tells us that we must live day to day and wait patiently for changes. Waiting is very hard. We'd like to take control and not just sit passively.

When we're with Daniel, Joel speaks loudly, hoping to penetrate this coma and bring him back to life.

"Daniel, wake up. You'll be late for school. Daniel, wake up now," he urges.

At home, our son would roll over and pull the blanket over his head. I'd love to hear him grumble again, "Go away, Dad. I've got a spare this morning."

Alyssa's approach is different. She's worried that if she asks him to do something that he cannot yet do, he may become frustrated and agitated, so she gently coaxes, "Daniel, when you're ready . . . Daniel, if you can."

Our daughter is a tower of strength with a core of optimism that bolsters us when our hopes begin to flag. When she returns to university on Sunday, Jonathan will be the only child left in the house. I think of him asleep in his room between ours and his brother's empty one. He's probably curled up with the teddy bear that he took down from the high shelf in his cupboard when he returned home today from David and Roz's. When Roz dropped him off after dinner, I rushed over to him and wrapped my arms around him, needing to feel his return hug, however brief.

"The house sure is quiet," Jonathan said, already missing the camaraderie of his cousins. He has not yet seen his brother.

At 4:30 a.m., I climb back into bed curling my body behind Joel's, my chest against his back, my knees pressed into his. He shivers and squirms. Without waking, he enfolds my right arm against his chest and holds it. I attune my breathing to his steady breath and slowly drift off to sleep.

CHAPTER FOUR

The rattling would start quietly and gradually increase until it was like the roar of a gorilla shaking the bars of its cage. What? Already? I glanced at my watch. Barely an hour had gone by, yet my seventeen-month-old son had already finished his nap. At his age, Alyssa used to sleep for at least two hours every afternoon, giving me some respite in the middle of the day. She'd awaken, gurgling and cooing and would play with her dolls, delighting in the movement of their eyes, their rigid eyelashes opening and closing when she tilted them up and down. Sometimes, when I came in to get her, she'd be hard at work undressing them, tiny plastic shoes pulled off and her fingers awkwardly tugging at pinafores fastened with Velcro.

Daniel was different. By the time I'd hurried upstairs and had flung open the door to his room, Teddy and his other stuffed animals were scattered about the floor, while there he stood, one leg raised high, trying to climb out of the crib by himself. Thank goodness Joel moved the mattress down to the lowest rung. Sensing deliverance, my caged son smiled sweetly at me, and as I reached to lift him up, he grabbed his fireman's hat from the crib post and plopped it on his head.

His diaper was dripping wet, but I carried him directly to the window, rather than to his changing table, and lifted the blind. Standing on top of his toy box, he eagerly looked outside. His whole body chuckled as he pointed to Sandy, our neighbour's golden retriever, lying on the front lawn across the street.

"Goggie, goggie," he squealed.

Squawks of protest followed when I insisted on changing his diaper and wet overalls. He squirmed on the dressing table like a wriggling monkey, and I had to pull him onto my lap on the floor to lace up his sneakers.

"Daniel, want some juice?" I asked.

Shaking his head from side to side, he pulled me towards the front door. A brief delay ensued while I inserted his arms into his red nylon jacket, emblazoned across the chest with a Little Sluggers emblem. Soon we were standing at the edge of our walkway, his hand firmly encased in mine. During the day there was seldom any traffic on our street, a quiet crescent cut off from the main thoroughfares by train tracks on one side and a ravine on the other.

"No cars, let's cross," I said after checking both ways.

Released onto the safety of the sidewalk, his arms pumped back and forth, the nylon jacket making swishing sounds, in time with his quickly paced steps. A boy with a purpose. He laughed as Sandy licked his face in greeting, and his hand bounced across her back, gently tugging on her long golden fur.

CHAPTER FIVE

On Thursday morning, September 2, four days after his operation, Joel and I watch Daniel open his eyes for the first time, and we hug each other with joy. How exciting! A signal of life and hope, although I'm reminded that it's just a reflex. We keep track of each positive sign — the bolt monitoring intracranial pressure was removed from his head and he's breathing now without a ventilator. Small steps . . . baby steps, but in the right direction.

Then back, too. When we visit in the afternoon, we find his face looking slack and his limbs heavy, motionless.

"A rise in heartbeat and blood pressure signalled the first concern," his nurse reports. "He appeared so agitated, thrashing his left arm and leg about, that the doctor prescribed a sedative."

Joel and I cannot anticipate the profound effect this news has on us. When we watch our son, it doesn't look so much like a sedation-induced sleep, but like death itself.

Soon after, we meet with a doctor to ask why Daniel's right arm and hand are puffed up to twice the natural size. He doesn't know this answer, but offers to explain the latest findings and the treatment plan. We find ourselves engulfed in medical terminology.

"The CAT scan shows no undue swelling of the brain or a shift of the midline, but there is still evidence of a haematoma. I expect the brain will reabsorb it on its own. Ultrasounds are scheduled for his legs to ensure that there are no blood clots that could potentially move to his lungs. We can't give him anti-coagulants because of the haematoma. A tracheotomy may be scheduled to replace the air tube in his mouth that the nurses are using for suctioning. Being a smaller tube, the trach tube is less prone to infection and inflammation."

Later, we realized that he was saying there was still a remnant of the blood clot that had been surgically removed early Monday morning. If the brain didn't reabsorb it as expected, would Daniel need more surgery? And what would happen if they discovered blood clots in his legs? We never got to ask those questions, overwhelmed as we were by the flow of information.

Back at home, I go into the kitchen and open the fridge, scanning the numerous casseroles that friends and family have provided. My stomach is so upset that I have little interest in food, but I take out a jar of chicken soup and rice.

"What would you like to eat?" I ask Joel.

"Nothing."

"Joel, you must eat something."

"What's the point?" His shoulders shudder. "Didn't you hear what the doctor said?"

"Yes, they're doing everything they can to ensure that Daniel will be okay." I hug him.

"But they can't guarantee it, can they?"

I turn away and heat our soup.

One day at a time . . . one day at a time. The days blend and blur into one another. By Friday, the words form a mantra I repeat over and over again. Our days have many empty hours and we don't know how to fill them. We're living in a state of time suspension with no concentration or interest in our usual activities. I haven't gone to work this week, and although Joel's been dropping by his office, it's as if he's pushing papers from one side of the desk to another. He phones home often to find out if there have been any reported changes.

All morning I pace around the house anxiously, phoning the hospital at twenty-minute intervals. I'm not allowed to visit. Finally, I get to speak to the nursing director, who informs me that Daniel has been put back on the ventilator following a restless night.

"The neurosurgeon would like to meet with you in an hour," she tells me.

My feelings swoop low, mirroring my son's setback. I phone Joel at his office and he tries to calm me down.

"I can come home right now if you'd like."

"No, I'm okay," I sniff as I pull another Kleenex from the package in my pocket. "I'll meet you there. Alyssa wants to come too."

The three of us wait in a small room. There's a nervous edge to our voices as we try to anticipate what the doctor will say. We had hoped that once the critical seventy-two-hour survival period had passed, things would go smoothly. To help pass the time, I flip open a magazine. The fashions may be five years out of date from the rumpled look of the cover, but I don't really care. Slowly, I turn the pages. Meanwhile, Joel paces from his seat to the door, peering down the hallway. Every ten minutes or so, he heads off to the payphone to make another call.

"Do you think she forgot about us?" I ask Alyssa. She checks with a nurse.

An hour and forty-five minutes go by.

Instead of the surgeon, in walks the resident, who had assisted in the surgery. He's tall, and when he folds his body into one of the chairs, his knees rise up high in front of him.

"The surgeon is busy in another emergency and asked me to talk to you." He leans forward towards us, eager to share the news.

"We're pleased with the success of the operation. We removed over 45 c.c.'s of blood from Daniel's brain."

We listen warily. We're becoming familiar with hearing bad news couched amidst the good.

The resident continues, "The Evoked Potential Tests, administered yesterday, suggest some neurological deficits, but their exact nature can't be determined. By your son's response to stimulation in all four limbs, it appears that he won't be paralysed on his right side."

We sigh with relief, unprepared for the bombshell about to be dropped.

The resident's long fingers drum on the arm of the chair. "Consciousness is considered a gradation of reactions. We know that he has started to open his eyes, but we aren't sure if he'll respond to his name or recognize family members. There are three levels of functioning, the third being social interactions and possible self-sufficiency. We expect that he has a very slim chance of reaching that level."

He stops speaking and smiles nervously, pleased as a young boy who has overcome stage fright in a school performance. Then he looks at his audience and becomes aware of the effect his message has on us. We try to remain composed, but our distraught expressions give us away.

"These remarks are gross predictions," he qualifies, but he can't take them back or undo the damage they've caused. When he leaves the room, I break down in tears, my hopes plummeting.

"Why did they save him? So that he could live in an institution or group home, perhaps being able to feed and dress himself, but not knowing his family or friends? What type of life did they save him for? Why'd they bother?"

Joel is crushed too as he hugs me in silence. The three of us walk out to the parking garage together. Joel returns to his office. As Alyssa drives me home, she tries to re-instil some hope. "Mom, Daniel is special. You know how strong he is. He'll be okay. You'll see."

How can I even visit Daniel if he senses my despair? I feel today that I have truly lost my son.

CHAPTER SIX

I awaken early on Saturday and head to the bathroom to pee and brush my teeth. The mirror reveals tousled hair and violet half-circles below my eyes. Taking off my glasses, I lean in for a closer look. The whites of my eyes are streaked with red lines like a child's crayon scribbles. It's no wonder I look like this. My sleep is so restless.

It's only 6:20 a.m. I tiptoe from the bedroom so I won't disturb Joel and I call the hospital. I want to speak to the night nurse before the shift changes at seven. Her information alarms me. Daniel has developed pneumonia and has been placed on three antibiotics. She has had to suction him frequently to clear his lungs. I feel drained and guilty. Did my words of despair yesterday make matters worse?

When Jonathan wakes up, I ask if he'll come with me to synagogue, and am surprised when he agrees. Sitting in the sanctuary, I try to turn off my fears about Daniel and concentrate on the service, while Jonathan tries his best to sit still beside me. My mother sits on his other side and gently strokes his arm. Her broad shoulders have become hunched with age yet still convey her resolute approach to any adversity. Stand tall and soldier on was the standard she and my father set in our family. What else would I expect from a former captain of the U.S. Women's Army Corps of wwii and a royal engineer of the Canadian Army?

The familiar words and melodies of the Sabbath service wash over me, but my gaze doesn't remain on the prayer book. Sunlight flickers through the stained glass windows and I follow the swaying branches of a linden tree, whose teardrop-shaped leaves shimmer like the tiny droplets that sneak from my eyes. On the wall beside me, brass memorial plaques catch the dancing sunlight.

Will my son's name join that wall?

I reflect on God and prayer. I don't believe in God responding to our personal prayers like a clerk filling a customer's order. But even if I did, what would I pray for — a speedy release from this nightmare of pain or the patience to endure a long-term and uncertain recovery? What would be better for Daniel?

When Joel and I visit Daniel in the afternoon, he is again so heavily sedated that we have a very short visit. His nurse informs us that Daniel is no longer on antibiotics. His white blood count is now fine and he has no fever. Can pneumonia disappear that quickly or was it misdiagnosed to begin with? Our confidence in the medical staff and their tests is shaken even as we're relieved by the news.

We hang around the house in the afternoon, with friends and relatives dropping by. Jonathan goes outside to play basketball with his cousins. The adults sit and talk, but we have nothing new to say. When my brother suggests going for a walk, I jump at the idea. Somehow it feels better to be moving.

The dog seems delighted, too. She's happy to trot along the familiar route through the neighbourhood. As we walk, I become aware of all the teenagers we pass playing road hockey, roller blading, and bike riding. Will Daniel ever be able to do any of these activities again? What will he be like? It's impossible to turn my mind off and refrain from contemplating unanswerable questions. I try to focus on Yaron's description of the latest play he's seen. I usually enjoy listening to his critiques; his tastes are closer to mine than the theatre critics in the newspapers. Today, he maintains a running monologue while I sometimes remember to interject a few meaningless words.

After dinner, Alyssa takes Jonathan for his first visit to Daniel. While they are gone, Joel and I stretch out in the family room to watch TV. We lie end-to-end on the long leather couch, our legs intertwined, and I cover myself with an afghan.

Click. Click. Three minutes of a science program, twenty seconds of a car commercial, then a sports event. Click. Click. Joel changes the channel again.

"Why can't you just leave it alone?" I ask.

"Is there anything you really want to watch?"

Just then the phone rings. He picks it up, his voice flat, almost toneless.

"Yes, still in coma. No, the doctors don't know." A mumbled, "No, nothing right now."

A familiar conversation that's been repeated many times over the past few days. Maybe we should just leave a taped message on our answering machine.

"Who was it?" I ask.

My husband's body seems to have taken on the sunken shape of the couch cushions. His voice sounds remote, as if waffling through a dense fog.

"John's father. He wanted to know how Daniel is, said how sorry they are and asked if there was anything they could do."

"What could they possibly do?"

"Nothing. I couldn't tell him what I really think, could I? How it should be his son lying in a hospital bed, not mine. Shit, it was John who was driving. It isn't fair."

Joel's eyes glare briefly at some point above my left shoulder and then soften as he turns to look directly at me. "Why does John get to walk out of the hospital after four days with nothing but a few scratches and a sore back? A sore back, big deal. And Daniel . . . ," his voice breaks.

I'm glad I wasn't the one who answered the phone. Our two sons are friends, but we've never met either of John's parents. As much as they sympathize, they must feel some sense of relief that it's not their son in a coma. That's the underlying message I'm imagining from everyone who calls. How awful! How tragic! But thank God it wasn't my child.

Alyssa and Jonathan return to find us sprawled in the dark, staring at a blank television screen. Blearily, Joel asks Jonathan how his visit went. Jonathan doesn't answer. Instead he reaches for his sister and lifts her over his shoulder, parading her around the room.

"Put me down," she giggles. "I'm not a canoe."

Laughing, he dumps her onto the other couch.

"I hope you're more gentle with the camp equipment," she admonishes.

"Don't worry, you're softer."

Jonathan flings himself onto her lap and she wraps her arms around him, hugging him. When he tries to squirm away, she tosses him over beside her and tickles him.

"Hey, stop that. No fair," he says, wriggling out of her reach.

Surprisingly, Joel and I laugh. It's so nice to realize we can still laugh.

My world has had its rhythm changed and I miss its familiar hum. In our quiet house we tiptoe around each other, afraid to bump into things. I miss the sound of Alyssa and her friends whose loud late-night whispers would be punctuated by giggles tinkling like bells. Now her giggle and Jonathan's squeal trigger memories of better times. Joel laughs quietly, his hee-hee-hee almost catching in the back of his throat, and my smile broadens when I see his eyes crinkle up, more the barometer of his pleasure than any loud guffaw.

I close my eyes and can picture the two of us lying contentedly on the couch at the cottage with our legs intertwined. Was it really ten years ago? I can still see the snow glistening on the balcony on the other side of the sliding glass doors and hear the children's laughter singing with the wind. Inside, the cottage felt snug and warm. My husband yawned and I replied with a deep wide sigh. We had spent hours outdoors that afternoon, walking down our cottage road to the fork at the end, then across another road to our favourite spot for tobogganing — a seldom used snowmobile trail on a narrow hillside dotted with skinny pine trees and bare maples. With one adult standing guard near the roadside, we trudged up the hill, each of us but the youngest taking turns pulling the long wooden toboggan. Then we settled down for the ride, hugging tightly to the body in front, the little one tucked into the middle so he wouldn't fall out.

Whoosh! The big push-off, then catching our breaths, leaning left, leaning right, trying to steer. Giggles and laughter as we zigged and zagged and bumped over the tree root stump in the middle of the pathway. The flat at the bottom slowed us down, the ride too soon ended.

After dinner, the children begged to go outside again to play, so we turned on the outside lights of the cottage, illuminating the darkened area near the kitchen window like a movie set. The lights reflected the glittery sparkles of snow, the scene a wintry wonderland. Like gophers popping out of a hole, the heads of the older two poked out now and then from a snow tunnel they were digging, while the youngest, wrapped snugly in his navy snowsuit and knitted hat, sat on top of a snow mound, intently licking beads of ice that were stuck to his mittens.

Droplets of water made icicles that cleaved to eavestroughs of my childhood home in Montreal, some icicles as large as stalactites I'd seen in pictures of caves. I remembered how my brothers and I used to stand on the stair ledge to knock them off, catching the smaller ones to lick like Popsicles and delighting when the larger ones shattered with loud crashing noises on the ground. Sometimes when the snow was deep, the icicle tips would sink right into the snow leaving the wide rough ends exposed, strange shapes for a winter garden. And when our street narrowed to a winding trail with parked cars buried in snow and jutting out at crazy angles, we'd dig out snow forts in the heavy snowbanks along the roadway and play inside them, gathering snowballs to fend off attacks from invaders. My mother read us newspaper reports of children crushed in snow forts when the plows came, but we thought those kids must have been stupid because everyone knew that snowplows make such noise you could hear them a block away.

Just thinking of crushed children made me get off the couch at the cottage to look out the kitchen window and check on the kids. Perhaps it was really the silence that disturbed me. For the moment, all three were quiet, lying on their backs — eyelashes dampened, darting tongues catching drifting snowflakes, and their arms sweeping up and down in the snow like angel wings. Soon enough the noise resumed. Rushing into the house with cheeks rosy red, they shed boots, hats, and mitts, peeled off snow pants and jackets that they heaped on the floor, then raced for the bathroom.

"I'm first!"

"No, me!"

Sounds are what I think of most. When they were younger, much of my sons' play was punctuated with noise: whoops, hollers, shrieks, and squeals of laughter that let me know where they were. Often after dinner, I would follow the sounds to the basement playroom.

"Yippee!"

Daniel had just scored. My husband stood sheepishly in net, his long arms and legs no longer moving everywhere at once. Bending down to retrieve the tennis ball, he tossed it out towards Jonathan. From the doorway, I watched my five-year-old son as he tried to stickhandle the ball that kept bouncing away. Joel waved off Daniel, who was eager to take it over and score again.

"You've got to give your brother a chance to play too, okay?"

When our younger son wound up for the shot, Joel lunged towards the right, making a large opening in the left side of the net. Surprised that the ball had reached its target, Jonathan dropped his plastic hockey stick and twirled about in delight trilling, "I scored! I scored!"

Daniel raced over and gave his brother a high-five, then winked at his father who raised an eyebrow in a noncommittal gesture. Soon the three of them were in a tussle on the floor, a squirming mass of arms and legs. Finally, Joel was pinned to the ground like Gulliver amid the Lilliputians, each son sitting on an arm. The loud sounds of play were somehow as reassuring to me as the crescendo of horns in a favourite symphony.

"We've got you this time, Dad."

"Not for long," Joel said, breaking free and snatching his younger son onto his lap for a hug. He stretched in vain for Daniel who laughed loudly, just out of reach.

CHAPTER SEVEN

As week two of Daniel's coma begins, Alyssa's room is a scene of organized chaos. She sits cross-legged on the floor, surrounded by boxes of books and bulging duffle bags. I'm on the edge of her bed, carefully buttoning her blouses before flipping them over to fold them — one sleeve, the other, and then in half, just like my Dad's work shirts when they had come packaged from the cleaners.

"Mom, you've got to listen. I don't want to go back to university now. I'll phone and defer my acceptance to the business program for a year."

I smooth the edge of a collar and add the shirt to the growing pile. "Alyssa, we've discussed this already. Daniel's life has been put on hold. We don't want yours to be too."

"But Mom, I should be here with you. You need me. Daniel needs me."

I sigh. In a way she's right. I'd love her to be here with us. She's mature enough to be involved in medical issues and such a support. I don't know where she finds her source for optimism; we're drawn to it like deer to a salt lick. But we don't want to lean on her. Besides, with our lives so drastically shaken, there seems to be an element of security in following plans.

"You need to go, Alyssa. Don't worry. We'll speak to you each day and you can come home every weekend."

I hand her the pile of blouses and she squeezes them into a duffle bag, creasing the edges as she zips the bag closed.

When I give my daughter a hug goodbye, I squeeze her tightly. She's so slim and her body feels so fragile, not sturdy and strong like Daniel's. What's to protect her? How can I let her go?

"You'll be fine," I promise, more to myself than to her. I'm glad she's not driving on her own this time. Joel is going to take her to her apartment in London, and with the help of his brother and our nephews, get her unpacked and set up.

After they leave, I visit Daniel and then go for a walk with Ellen and another friend in the ravine. Away from the noise of the streets, I feel transported to another time and place. The path winds beside a bubbling stream and meanders through the woods. I can sense the stillness amid the greenery and waters. Grumff. The croak of a frog and then the answering call of another. I watch the sweep of a bird's wings as it hovers over the bog and then gracefully alights on a fallen log. The frogs disappear. A rising mist gently covers the silken threads of a spider's web on a birch branch. Without any warning, my internal video starts to play. Superimposed on this peaceful scene is the picture of my son lying in his hospital bed. My breath becomes shallow and my eyes brim with tears.

"Sorry, I must go."

When Ellen asks if I'd like her to come too, I shake my head, accept her hug, and rush back to the hospital.

Later that afternoon, Roz is with me when the neurosurgeon comes over to speak. The doctor wants to clarify the negative impression her resident gave us on Friday. "I believe that Daniel's youth will aid in his recovery," she says hopefully. "However, I'd advise you not to seek any long-term prognosis at this stage."

School starts on Tuesday, September 8. I go in to visit Daniel at 7:00 a.m. and return home by the time Jonathan is in the kitchen for breakfast.

"Cold cereal? Mom, could you make me French toast tomorrow?"

I ruffle his hair. I'm worried about him. On Sunday, he didn't want to go with Joel to drive Alyssa to university even though his two cousins were going. And yesterday, when Ellen and her husband Marc dropped in, Ellen commented that Jonathan seemed unusually quiet. The phone had been ringing so often with calls of support from our friends that I hadn't even noticed. Now that I think about it, I realize that Jonathan must have spent the whole day in the basement watching TV, instead of going out to play ball or go bike riding with friends.

"Do you want a lift to school?" I ask.

"Naw. I'm meeting Jordan."

"How about after school? Should I pick you up on my way to the hospital?"

Lowering his eyes, Jonathan mumbles, "What do you expect me to say to him? He can't hear me anyway."

When Jonathan leaves for school, I crawl back into bed fully dressed. Joel has said he'd like to be able to go to sleep for a month and not have to live with all this uncertainty and waiting. We've put on a façade of strength, but the cracks are so evident. Already I miss Alyssa.

Ten minutes later, I force myself out of bed and drive to work. My leather briefcase, almost empty, feels so heavy in my hand. I pull open the door and enter the school board office. The receptionist smiles at me as she answers the phone and jots down a message. Mouthing a silent hello, I follow the tapping sounds of computer keys and the beep of a fax machine to the main office where the secretaries greet me. Their compassionate looks tell me that they've already heard the news about Daniel. There is little to say. I open the top drawer of the filing cabinet and check my file.

"Look at all these cases," I say, pulling out a stack of student referrals. "I'd better get started."

My desk is removed from the main activity area, and today I welcome its seclusion. I try to do some reading and note taking. Somehow time passes. Jim, my supervisor, comes in to talk. His eyes share his concern, although his formal manner allows just a dry handshake.

"I want you to take it easy. Would you like me to inform the schools for you?"

"No thanks, I'll handle it."

"Let me know if you need anything."

I take a deep breath and phone the first of six special education representatives at my schools. After the usual pleasantries are exchanged, I tell her about my son. Eileen is supportive and caring.

"Oh, how awful. Don't worry about the testing. The students will still be here when you're ready."

On Wednesday morning, I attend a committee meeting with some of my colleagues from the psychology department. When I enter the meeting room, everyone looks relaxed and well rested from the summer vacation. A few people are milling around the coffee table, filling their cups and chatting; the rest are already seated at the table.

"So how was your summer? What did you do?" someone asks cheerily as I pour myself a cup of tea.

My body stiffens and my face becomes masklike. Like a robot, I begin to tell Daniel's story. My colleagues gather around me, their carefree smiles suddenly displaced. One of them gives me a hug and my tears are released, trickling out despite my efforts to control them. Are tears contagious? Several of my colleagues need to wipe their eyes too. We share sniffles and a box of tissues.

"Would anyone like to start the meeting?" I ask.

We take our seats and settle down to business. The discussion starts off slowly with suggestions carefully tendered. As the meeting proceeds, voices become more animated as points are bounced back and forth like a tennis ball slamming into the far side of the court. My pad of paper sits blankly in front of me. When I empty my tea, I'm surprised to find heavily inked lines etched and shaded into the Styrofoam cup. I excuse myself and leave the meeting early.

It's more than a thirty-minute drive back to the hospital. Midway, I can sense a tightness pulling across my shoulders. My fingers are gripping the steering wheel, clenched like a dog's teeth around a bone. I release one hand, shake it out, and then do the same with the other.

At the hospital, I drive up the ramp to the garage and stretch sideways to take a parking ticket from the dispenser. There's a light honk behind me. Checking my rearview mirror, I see Joel just pulling in. He smiles and waves. We find spots close to one another.

"How come you're here? I thought you had a meeting," Joel asks as he bends over to give me a kiss.

"I left early. What about you?"

"I was just heading back to my office so I thought I'd drop in."

Joel is lucky that his office is located in midtown Toronto near the hospital, instead of downtown like so many of the other chartered accountancy firms. I wish I worked closer too.

We ride the elevator up to the seventh floor visitor's lounge, where I smile at the silver-haired volunteer. She recognizes us, and without being asked, phones the unit to request permission for us to visit Daniel. Shaking her head, she replaces the receiver, "He isn't there."

My hand reaches for Joel's in a panic.

"What do you mean?" Joel rasps.

"It's okay," she says quickly. "He's been moved to the neurological intensive care unit on the fifth floor."

Joel and I bound down the two flights of stairs, Joel taking several steps at a time. The waiting room here is much smaller and has no volunteer. My husband follows the instructions posted on the wall to call into the unit, but we have to wait about thirty-five minutes before the nurse phones back, permitting us to see our son.

Daniel's internal thermostat is out of kilter. Rivulets of sweat pour from him. He looks like he just came out of a shower without towelling off. I watch a nurse dip a cloth into ice water, wring it out, and then wipe him. New rivers of sweat immediately form on his brow.

"I can do this," I say, wishing to be useful. There is so little I can do for my son other than sitting by his bedside. I talk to him, and when I can no longer think of words to say, I read to him from the latest John Grisham novel, which he had brought home from camp. Daniel will now often open his eyes when we are there, and his heartbeat shoots up. We believe that he senses our presence even if he is not fully conscious or aware. The nurses become concerned when he's agitated, but I can sense the life that still throbs within him when he's moving. I find it harder to watch him when he's restful.

As I wipe his forehead, I notice a bulge over his left eyebrow. His nurse warns us that he's scheduled for another CAT scan. The doctors are worried about hydrocephalus, fluid on the brain. If they're right, he'll need a shunt to drain it. One more thing to worry about.

In the midst of all this, my friend Karen offers to go grocery shopping for me, but the thought of figuring out which items I need is overwhelming. It seems easier to do it myself and I'm grateful for the normalcy that this task represents. I drive Jonathan to the mall to buy school supplies and pick up some groceries. Do we look like any other mother and son on an outing? Jonathan has grown over the summer and is now a few inches taller than I am. His long legs carry him along at a quicker pace than mine. I worry about where they'll take him.

We follow the teachers' lists and purchase new notebooks and binders. I expect that soon they'll be scruffy-looking and covered in doodles; today the bright colours look fresh.

At the supermarket, I feel besieged by the vast array of choices. With little appetite, it's hard for me to find any food appealing, but my son cheerfully fills the cart as he pushes it up and down the aisles. He zigs and zags from one side to the other, making me dizzy. Then he reaches up to a high shelf and grabs a box of crackers. Spinning around, he slam dunks the box into our basket, exclaiming, "Michael Jordan, watch out."

CHAPTER EIGHT

Thursday, day eleven, and there's no change in Daniel's condition. We're marking time, crossing off each day from the calendar like survivors who've been shipwrecked or kidnapped. We keep hoping for rescue, waiting for his coma to lift. The longer it lasts, the worse the prognosis. At least that's how it seems to us. No one is prepared to contradict this theory, although friends ply us with stories of people they've heard about — some guy from the bowling league or some woman at work, a neighbour, a cousin — the list seems endless. I've never heard of so many people who've had brain injuries. Yet it seems that no two are alike and my son's injury sounds more severe than any of the others.

We have no one to compare him to in the hospital. Most of the patients in the neurological intensive care unit are older people who've had strokes. One day a visitor, a man in his thirties, overheard me talking to Joel and interrupted us.

"Excuse me," he said. "Your friends are right. I'm living proof. Don't give up hope."

My mother gathers her strength and comes to stand with me by Daniel's bedside. Her lips quiver as she stares down at her eldest grandson. When I place my arm around her waist, she brushes it off, not wanting me to feel her shaking body.

Two of her sisters have flown in from New York to add their support. Doris, who is a school librarian, croons songs to my son, songs I used to sing to him when he was young. Where is he? Returned to his childhood or continuing on to adulthood? We don't know.

My mother, my aunts, and I walk over to K-Wing to visit my father. The elevator door opens directly onto the lounge where a game show blares on the large-screen TV. One veteran sits moaning in his wheelchair, his trunk held in place by a thick white strap that encircles his chest, his pant legs pinned back above where his knees used to be. As we walk by, he points to the tiled floor and shouts, "Watch out for the mines. Don't step on those land mines."

I hold my breath as we pass through the haze of cigarette smoke wafting through the lounge. The hallway to my father's room is little better, with its strong smell of disinfectant masking the odour of stale urine.

My father is lying on his bed dressed in blue sweatpants and a green sweatshirt. He never used to wear sweatsuits. When I was young, he'd leave for work looking the part of the professional notary, dressed in a tailored suit, white shirt, and carefully knotted tie. Even his casual clothes had crispness to them.

"Dad, how'd you like to go downstairs for some coffee?" I ask.

"Sure," he says, putting down yesterday's newspaper. He turns to one of his roommates, "Goodbye. My mother has come to take me home now."

I can tell that my mother is upset by the way she fusses over Dad, urging him to hurry, even offering to tie up his shoelaces as her sisters wait outside the room. When my father is finally ready, we pass back through the smoky lounge and wait for the elevator. Two of the veterans are playing a game of cards. "Son-of-a-bitch, you're a lucky bastard," one says as he throws down his hand. His opponent's hands tremble as he gathers the cards to shuffle and deal another round.

We match our pace to my father's slow shuffle. At the cafeteria counter, Dad orders pie and coffee. He pats his back pocket looking for his wallet, then his front pockets both left and right. His face takes on a look of consternation.

"Don't worry, Dad. It's my treat today."

"What a nice daughter," he says.

He doesn't notice my sadness and anxiety; I don't tell him about Daniel's injury. He wouldn't understand or remember.

I used to love watching my father swim. He'd carefully tuck his glasses into the pocket of his beach top before folding it neatly on the bench, then he'd stride to the end of the pier, his hairless legs flashing white as he dived. With smooth, even strokes, he'd swim effortlessly from the dock, parallel to the shoreline. He never seemed to tire. When he waded back to the beach, my younger brother Peter and I would call out and wave to him. But without his glasses on, he'd look towards shore confused, trying to make out those strange creatures on the beach — perhaps not really his children, after all.

Each summer, my parents rented a cottage in a community in the Laurentians, north of Montreal, and every morning the mothers would gather up all the kids with pails and shovels held tightly in hand, herding us across the road to the beach. My mom pushed my youngest brother Stevie in a carriage, the tray underneath filled with our towels and snacks as well as his bottles and diapers. At the lake was a pier where the mothers could relax on wooden benches and supervise our play. Peter and I spent hours with the other children digging in the sand, making mud pies, moats, and sand castles topped with pinecones or acorns. Racing to the water, we'd stop knee-deep and fill our pails, sloshing them against our sides as we trudged back with our heavy loads. If a child seemed too daring and ran further out into the water, some mother would call, "Come back, now." It didn't matter whose child it was.

When it was very hot, the mothers waded into the lake up to their thighs or waist, gently splashing water on their arms, the back of their necks, and their chests, where droplets would dribble down into the fronts of their bathing suits. Real swimming was reserved for the weekends, after the fathers came up Friday nights from the city. The blowing dust on the road swirled and scattered through the trees, urgent smoke signals announcing the men's arrival. Then higgledy-piggledy they'd emerge from their cars as if from alien spaceships, white shirt collars unbuttoned, jackets slung over their left elbow, right arms crooked and loaded with parcels, maybe a fresh *challah* or bagels from a bakery in Montreal.

"Daddy, Daddy," we'd call, and the weeklong stranger would put down his packages and twirl us around.

On Saturday morning after my father's swim, I got my turn. He promised to catch me when I held my breath and let my body lie still in a dead man's float — and he did. But he couldn't get me to turn my head to the side and blow bubbles the way he did. I kept swallowing water.

When my children were young, we too spent time each summer at a cottage. Our first place was right on a river with a large sandy beach where birches and poplars grew close to the bank. Across the narrow river, a large oak tree leaned partway to one side as if bending over to say hello. The water was always dark there, murky from the rotting leaves that lined the riverbed, and along the shoreline tall weeds grew, thin strands of swaying green, and sometimes flat lily pads bobbed on the river's surface. With butterfly nets, my kids became adept at catching minnows that darted in and out of those waving fronds. When they weren't catching toads and minnows, they spent hours in the sand with their shovels and pails, filling their buckets for sand castle moats, the water runnelling through channels and overflowing the banks. Alyssa, in charge, would squeal at her brother to get fresh mud to patch up the leaks.

I remember Joel swimming in the water with Alyssa and my father teaching Daniel how to float. "Danielfish," we called him. He loved the water so much that we had to drag him out each time, shivering and blue-lipped. My mother or I would wrap him in a towel, rubbing him warm.

It wasn't until I was thirty-one years old and pregnant with Jonathan that I finally learned how to swim front crawl. Unable to continue with regular exercise classes, I enrolled in private swim lessons. The clerk at the registration desk wanted me to sign up for a full series of eight lessons, but when I backed away from the counter and she saw my expanded belly, she quickly agreed that four would be quite enough.

The day of my first lesson, I eased myself down the steps of the pool and demonstrated what I could do, traversing the length of the pool with sidestroke and backstroke, like someone balancing a big beach ball on top of her tummy. I wasn't afraid of deep water. I just wasn't happy putting my face in it. Then the instructor asked me to swim front crawl. Gulping and gurgling, I spewed out water each time I turned my head to the side and tried to breathe. After watching me struggle for half a length, she allowed me to stand and suggested that next time I equip myself with nose plugs, goggles, and a bathing cap. Surprisingly, they helped.

When our youngest was a year old, we sold our small riverfront place and bought a larger cottage on a lake that had only deepwater access. At first, Jonathan was content to play beside me on the dock that Joel reinforced with struts like a playpen to make sure he couldn't fall in. We'd fill his inflatable pool with pails of hot water that we lugged down from the cottage, and sometimes Alyssa and Daniel would sit with him in the warm pool, splashing and playing.

I knew it wouldn't be long before he'd graduate from it and would want to join his brother and sister cavorting in the lake with their dad. At age three, he'd float on his back with a lifejacket on, kicking his feet as I pulled him over to the black inner tube where Joel hovered nearby the raft. With Jonathan safe in his father's arms, I would take my turn to swim.

Red and yellow hula-hoops floated in the water invitingly. Our kids dived ceaselessly, asking us to grade them from one to ten like scorers in a sports event. Alyssa, always so graceful, soared in the air before slicing through the water in the middle of a hoop, emerging with her long hair streaming down her back.

"Ten," Joel said and Jonathan clapped.

Then Daniel dived, his form perfect until the moment of contact when he'd cross his feet, hooking his toes together.

"Eight. Good try."

"Mom, you watch me this time," he said, scrambling back onto the raft. "You'll see. I'll get it."

And he tried and he tried, again and again — until his teeth chattered and his lips turned blue, until we forced him back onto land.

CHAPTER NINE

Week three begins with a different beat. Unlike the muted shuffle of the nursing staff's crêpe soles, the tapping of fine leather heels announces the presence of the social worker as she approaches the waiting room.

"How are you doing?" she asks with concern, noting my blotchy red nose and the droop in our shoulders.

"Coping," I reply, straightening my slouched posture. "At least I think we are."

She sits down in the chair across from us and places her binder on her lap. She has an elegant look that seems out of place in this hospital setting. Her makeup is carefully done and her hair is coiffed, unlike mine. When I put on lipstick earlier today, I noticed my bangs straggling over my eyes.

"How's Daniel?" she asks.

"Well, his eyes are open more and he turns his head sometimes, but he still doesn't respond to any commands."

She nods her head sympathetically. "And the other children?"

"Seem okay. Back in school. We speak to Alyssa every day."

"That's good. And you? You can't spend all your time in the hospital."

"I've gone back to work."

Her eyebrows lift, suggesting that this announcement is unexpected and perhaps unwise.

Then her gaze turns to my husband, who sits silently next to the phone — staring at it, willing it to ring.

"Did you know that a lot of marriages break up from this kind of stress? You've got to let go of it somehow. When was the last time you two did something together?"

Joel shifts his eyes and glares at her, daring her to continue. I'm annoyed too. What does she expect? Her words feel so out of place, like someone trying to teach a drowning person how to swim instead of tossing out a life preserver. We're so concerned about Daniel right now. Are we supposed to worry about the state of our marriage too?

Just then the phone rings. Joel grabs it and cocks his head in the direction of the neurological intensive care unit. He stands and waits for me.

The social worker fumbles with her binder. "I'll check on you in a few days," she says, reaching her hand forward as if to pat me on my shoulder. Instead she lifts it and fluffs a wayward curl back in place. Her heels clickety-clack as she leaves the lounge.

We're pleased to see that Daniel's eyes are open, but disturbed that he's quite agitated. His left knee is bent and moving rapidly; his left hand, clenched in a fist, rubs against his stomach. When I take hold of his hand, his T-shirt lifts, revealing an ugly purple bruise just under his ribs.

"C'mon, cutie, it's okay," I cajole, trying to pry his fingers apart. He feels warm to my touch and is sweating profusely. Joel takes the washcloth from the basin behind his bed and wipes Daniel's forehead. His voice is gentle.

"Daniel, when you were five or six, you used to get into such mischief. One day I came home from work and found clumps of mud everywhere. Splattered against the siding above the garage and splotched on the roof. I looked around. Then I noticed two sets of muddy footprints on top of Mom's station wagon. Uh, oh! Daniel and Daniel had struck again. You and your pal, Daniel, from across the street were terrors together. Remember him? Was I ever happy when his family moved to Calgary."

Joel dips the cloth in the ice water again and wrings it out. "Daniel, we've helped you every time you got into trouble. We're going to help you get through this too."

Passing the lounge on our way out, we hear a familiar voice calling us. I look into the room anticipating Daniel's friend Matt, with his mop of unruly blond curls. I'm surprised to find three other guys sitting there with him, lined up in a row like patients in a dentist's office. The boys' teenage exuberance is held in check in this serious setting and one of them rhythmically taps his foot. Blond, dark, dark, blond. Four heads all smiles, nervous smiles. Only Matt's seems genuine.

One part of me is grateful that the boys are here, while another part wonders whether they're just looking to satisfy their own curiosity like the nursing director implied when we met with her last Thursday. We wanted to get permission for Daniel's friends to visit so we approached her, a thin-faced woman whose grey eyes seemed to pierce right through us. She gazed around the room, ensuring that everything was in order before directing her attention back to us.

"I'm sorry, the rules include only extended family members."

"We know, but we believe that he may respond to his friends. We'd like to try."

"This request is highly unusual."

My voice took on an imploring tone. "You don't understand. To a seventeen-year-old, his peers are his life. More important in many ways than immediate family."

Her pursed lips softened, "Are you sure that you want him seen this way? It's pretty degrading to be wearing a diaper."

"The guys will understand. They've been making tapes for him of his favourite music and telling him stories about school, hockey, and camp. They need to be here. Daniel would want them to be here."

Turning in dismissal, she headed back to the nursing station. "I'll consider this and let you know."

Now his friends are here. I smile warmly at them. The boys ask about Daniel and we try to prepare them for what they'll see: his shaved head, the tubes and machines. I don't know how they'll react.

Matt breaks through my scepticism.

"I saw him last night. Tubes, machines, so what? He's still Daniel."

"How's school going?" I ask, reluctant to leave although I feel Joel's pull on my sleeve. They're all in their final year of high school, as our son would have been.

"Just started, but seems okay."

"A lot of the kids are asking about Daniel. They'd like to visit."

"So would his grade twelve English teacher. She says she'll get in touch with you."

Once again the red numbers on the bedside clock inform me that it's not quite 6:00 a.m. My husband is curled up in a fetal position breathing deeply; I know I won't fall back to sleep again. Lying on my back, I consider my options. It's too early to go to work or visit the hospital. My library book sits unread on my night table, while yesterday's newspaper still lies folded on the front hall table, not even taken into the kitchen. I no longer have any interest in current events and won't turn on the radio or television for news. Too many people dying in events both natural and man-made. I don't want to know about them.

You may as well resume your studying, I tell myself, like some theatrical director offering advice to an actor who hasn't yet captured the desired effect. This suggestion seems so preposterous it has the power to propel me out of bed to the spare bedroom down the hall that doubles as my home office. On the coffee table sits the stack of eight thick study guides that I haven't looked at since Daniel's injury two weeks ago.

At a staff meeting last spring, we learned that the College of Psychology was opening a new category for professionals with Master-level degrees who had completed five years of supervised training. If we passed the same rigorous tests that the doctoral candidates took, we could apply for membership in the College as Psychological Associates and practise autonomously. Many members of my department expressed interest, for the notion of not having all our reports read by a supervisor was appealing. However, only two of us proceeded directly with the plans. During the summer when I was off work, I spent every morning studying. With this concentrated focus, I had expected to be well prepared for the four-hour long written exam scheduled for mid-October. At the end of August, I had been covering the section on neuropsychology and the functions of the different parts of the brain.

Now because of my son, I'm getting first-hand knowledge. I wish I wasn't.

I pick up one of the study manuals. It feels heavy in my lap. Opening it, I flip past the chapter on neuropsychology and start reading. My eyes scan the words and my fingers grip a yellow highlighter, marking what should be key phrases. I don't know if I'm absorbing anything. I find myself reading the same paragraph again and again.

When 7:00 a.m. comes, I go downstairs, phone the hospital to check on Daniel — still no change — and then make some French toast for Jonathan's breakfast. While waiting for the griddle to heat, I place the study guide in my briefcase, something to read during school recess if I don't want to go into the staff room. I feel better with this plan of action. It helps to counteract my feelings of helplessness.

Work does the same. It feels good to smile and encourage the youngsters I work with. To assess students with learning difficulties, I must observe and listen, put away my own problems to help solve theirs. My professional demeanour enables me to block feelings about my son that threaten to engulf me. How close to the surface those feelings lie.

After a lunchtime meeting, the teachers hurry back to class. The special education administrator, whom I know well, lingers. When she asks me how I'm doing, I burst into tears.

"You must continue to have faith and hope," Cathy says, giving me a hug.

"How?" I ask. "Where do faith and hope come from?"

I see these qualities in others and I'm envious. One woman in the visitor's lounge is always so cheerful and hopeful. I don't know how she does it. Doesn't she understand? Her twenty-nine-year-old husband fell forty-five feet out of a tree that he was cutting. He has already had five operations to fix his shattered elbow and he's still in a coma. She was just told yesterday that he has only a fifty-fifty chance of coming out of the coma at all, and if he does he will be dependent upon her for the rest of his life.

"We'll just take each day as it comes," she says, a philosophy of life that seems so elusive to me.

Joel and I have prided ourselves on living our lives effectively according to five-year plans. Degrees, work, travel, children — everything planned, under control, and successful too. How can we learn to wait for things to unfold? One day at a time . . . it seems impossible.

CHAPTER TEN

The Jewish New Year arrives. Joel would just as soon ignore the holiday and spend the time in the hospital, but we've always gotten together with family. When the children were young, we used to drive into Montreal to be with our relatives. I used to dread those long car rides. It wasn't the anxious expectation about visiting family; I quite looked forward to that. Showing off our kids and having them spoiled by two sets of grandparents for a few days was quite a treat. It was the drive itself that filled me with trepidation.

It wasn't so bad before we had kids. It didn't matter then that the landscape was flat and monotonous. Joel liked to drive. We'd turn on the radio and talk, nibbling on the sandwiches and fresh fruit I'd packed, my hand often resting on his thigh. When the radio signal developed too much static, I'd turn the dial, seeking something other than country music, then settle for silence that allowed us to drift into comfortable reverie. Joel didn't even mind if I picked up a book and read for an hour or so. Time would whiz by with just one quick pit stop. But with kids, that scenario changed.

I was always stuck with the job of keeping the children quiet and entertained — not an easy task, since our daughter tended to get carsick after a thirty-minute drive and Daniel hated to be restrained. The first problem was solved through experimentation: we learned to give Alyssa a light dose of anti-nausea syrup mixed in with some strawberry flavouring in a glass of milk before each long trip. She looked forward to this unusual treat of strawberry milk and could keep herself amused for hours with her dolls, books, and colouring.

Daniel was another story. His limit for the car seat was twenty minutes. Then he'd squirm, whine, and pull at the straps, trying to get out and move around. Not quite Houdini, he hadn't yet mastered his own escape and the seatbelt remained firmly secured around him. Like a magician with a bag of tricks, I tried to forestall the inevitable by pulling out toys to distract him — his teddy bear, a plastic car, and a squeaking rubber duck. Becoming an actor, I'd growl, vroom, and quack as one by one the toys bounced through the air and onto his lap, before ending up on the floor.

After the toys came the treats. But how many Cheerios, crackers, or cookies is a mother prepared to give without worrying about stomachaches or other complications? Too many bottles of liquid meant an extra pit stop for a diaper change and then it was imposs-ible to strap him back in. Released from the car seat restraints, Daniel would pull away from my hold while I tugged on the straps of his overalls to keep him upright and balanced. Sometimes he'd stand quietly in his car seat looking out the back window at the moving cars behind us and surprisingly, he'd settle down on my lap when Alyssa swirled her small fingers in circles on his pudgy arm.

Then from my bottomless bag, I'd extract some books, first a Dr. Seuss book for Daniel and then Alyssa's favourite, *The Story of Ping*. No matter how many times she'd heard the story, she'd cringe when poor Ping was captured and threatened with being turned into duck stew.

"Mommy, quick, turn the page to where Ping escapes."

Joel seemed miles away with his attention fixed on the road and the traffic, as if there were a heavy sheet of glass — like in a taxi in New York or London — separating him from the commotion in the back.

I remember how, one time, I ran through my repertoire, singing Raffi songs and old army tunes my parents had taught us, before Alyssa drifted off to sleep. Meanwhile Daniel, still awake, tapped the pages of his book, a relentless taskmaster. As we pulled off the expressway, he finally dozed off and missed the ten-minute drive through the streets of Montreal to my parents' home.

I grew up in this house, a semi-detached bungalow, with mounds of spiraea plants hugging the front stairs. Alyssa raced up the concrete steps and bounded into her grandmother's arms while my father gave me a hug. The vestibule was crowded and we moved aside quickly to make way for Joel, carrying a heavy child in his arms. He strode directly down the hall to my old bedroom where a crib had been set up.

"What can I get you?" my mother asked. "Some fresh apple cake? Or, maybe you'd like some of the chocolate Danish I bought for Joel. I'll put on the kettle."

I followed the scent of cinnamon into the kitchen and slumped into one of the bucket-shaped blue chairs, swivelled around to look at the Scrabble board filled with snaking letters and at the rack of tiles where someone had arranged a seven-letter word. There was no opening on the board for it.

Alyssa headed to the dining room, where a small red table awaited her, covered with paper, crayons, a stapler, an old calculator with a paper tape, and gold seals from my father's notarial office for deeds of sale.

"Hey Papa, my office is still here. Sit down and I'll make you something," Alyssa said, gesturing to one of the two kid-sized metal chairs.

Just as the kettle boiled, fresh wails erupted from down the hall. Daniel wasn't sleeping after all. My mother offered to run water in the bath, squirting in some bubble bath from a yellow container shaped like Big Bird from Sesame Street, while I undressed my sobbing son. The whole bathroom engulfed us in yellow: fixtures, tiles, even the curtains, bath mat, and towels.

The warm water soothed him and he squealed with delight as his rubber ducky swooped and dived through the bubbles. Kneeling beside the deep tub, I scrubbed his body, remembering shared baths in this tub with my brother, our shampooed hair spiked in peaks like the wings of a duck ready to soar.

The first evening of this Rosh Hashanah, I convince my husband to go to his brother's home for dinner, after promising that we'll have time to visit Daniel. Joel's mother has come into town. It's the first holiday celebration since his father died, and she's fresh with grief for both the loss of her husband and the injury to her grandson. Joel and I are so caught up in our own pain, we have little comfort to offer her.

My sister-in-law, Roz, lights the holiday candles, and David recites the blessings over the wine and the *challahs* that are flecked with raisins, their circular shape a symbol of the wholeness of life. When we dip slices of apples into honey and say a blessing, wishing each other a sweet New Year, Daniel's absence from the dinner table is even more pronounced than my late father-in-law's.

After dinner, Alyssa invites her *Bubbie* to sit beside her on the couch, removing her from the bustle of clearing the table and cleaning up. As the eldest grandchild and only granddaughter, my daughter has a special place in her *Bubbie*'s heart. Alyssa's light brown curls lean towards her grandmother's white ones as they whisper like two schoolgirls with secrets to share.

Standing at the sink, I clear off the dirty plates and stack them on the counter. David loads them into the dishwasher while Roz covers the leftovers and places them in the fridge. Joel leans against the door. He's too edgy to sit and too distracted to help. Peals of laughter emerge from the basement — Jonathan and his cousins are playing ping-pong and roughhousing. My nephews' dog, Scamper, joins the tumult with her yaps of protest. When Alyssa notes her father's distress, she offers to drive Jonathan home so we can leave for the hospital.

The next evening, my brother Yaron, his wife Sue, and my mother join us for the second night of the holiday. I take out my camera and invite everyone to the living room for our customary family pictures. Alyssa and Jonathan line up in front of the fireplace and beckon Joel to take his place with them.

Joel protests, "How can you even think of taking family photos that don't include Daniel?"

"Joel, please," I say. "We have pictures of every holiday in our albums. One day Daniel will be with us again. He may want a record of this time that he's missing."

We soon arrive at a compromise and move away from the fire-place. Yaron takes one shot of us as a couple and the next of Alyssa and Jonathan with their grandmother. Then we gather around the dining room table, repeating the same rituals performed the night before.

I'd spent hours in the kitchen preparing many of our favourite dishes to mark the celebration of the New Year. When I diced onions, my eyes teared as usual, but they kept on streaming as I grated potatoes, measured out matzo meal, and beat eggs for the potato *kugel*. Would anyone notice the extra-salty flavouring in it this year? I carry in a platter of salt and pepper gefilte fish with tangy horse-radish. Next comes the simmering chicken soup with *knadlach*, fluffy matzo balls that float just below the golden surface. My mother contributes *tsimmis*, her usual carrot, prune, and pineapple dish and her famous meatballs, which are Daniel's favourite. He always wolfed them down and asked for seconds. When I'd warn him to save room for the turkey, sweet noodle pudding, and other side dishes, he'd laugh, reassuring me that meatballs didn't count, they slid down so quickly.

During dinner, I notice the clang of cutlery against the china plates. It's hard to find neutral subjects to talk about and we don't want to talk about Daniel. My brother asks the kids questions about their classes. Alyssa responds, but Jonathan remains as silent as his father has been throughout the meal. By the time I serve Sue's fruit platter and honey cake for dessert, Joel looks like he's been held together by string that has slowly unravelled. Excusing himself, he lies down in the family room. Covered from head-to-toe with a crocheted afghan, he looks like a mummy wrapped in green wool. Our relatives don't linger. When the dishwasher is loaded, Jonathan retreats to the basement to watch television. Alyssa and I return to the hospital to visit Daniel.

CHAPTER ELEVEN

The heat of summer has waned and without consciously registering the change, I've started wearing sweaters in the evening to combat the nip in the air. It's been three weeks now since Daniel's injury and I haven't been aware of much that's around me, so focussed am I on my son. As my car pulls out of the driveway, I see that the geraniums in our front garden have become leggy. I haven't dead-headed the faded blooms and the dried-up black circles now out-number the blooming pink flowers. Don't know when I'll get to them.

I'm exhausted and distressed by this endless waiting.

After three days of scheduling and cancellation, Daniel finally has a tracheotomy procedure to insert a tube directly into his windpipe to aid in breathing. We were getting concerned because he didn't receive any nourishment during the time prior to the expected surgery. Late in the day, when the nurses knew for certain that he wasn't going to be operated on, they'd hook up his feeding tube again.

It's so nice to see his face again without so many tubes. But is it just my imagination, or has he already lost weight? I run my fingers along his sharply angled cheekbones and down the side of his face to the cleft in his chin. His bronzed skin has paled to a ghastly pallor and his eyes, when open, have a vacant stare.

I experience mixed feelings — relief that the procedure went well, continued anxiety about the lack of noticeable change.

Joel and I are just about to leave the unit when a sandy-haired physician approaches us. When he extends his right hand to introduce himself, his voice is warm and welcoming like an old-fashioned doctor, the kind from the seventies TV shows who used to make house calls and knew everyone's names, even the family dog's.

"I've been asked to look over your son's chart because his neurosurgeon is going to be leaving the hospital soon. You may have heard already that she has a new position in the States."

He lifts up the file in his hand, but doesn't open it. His voice becomes guarded, his eyes hooded, his expression almost pained, "The prognosis for your son isn't very good, I'm afraid. The frontal lobe and left hemisphere of the brain sustained significant trauma. Motor deficits on the right side of the body are severe enough to render that side of the body non-functional, and I expect he'll have other deficits as well."

"What do you mean?"

"I don't expect your son will be able to walk or talk again."

"Well, if he can't talk he'll just have to communicate through writing," I say, picturing several students I've seen with alternative communication devices. The most sophisticated are computers with voice-activated output attached to their wheelchair trays.

"I'm afraid you don't understand," the physician replies. "The section of his brain that was injured affects the entire language area. That means more than just not talking. It infers an inability to make sense of symbols that would affect both reading and writing."

Joel and I fall silent.

"I'm concerned about his receptive language skills as well. Re-habilitation will be tied to his ability to understand the instructions given by a physiotherapist or occupational therapist. He may not have the capability for learning new skills or even relearning old ones."

In a stunned state, we leave the unit and make our way back to our car. I use the car phone to call Ellen and when we arrive at her home, the three of us go for a walk in the nearby ravine. For over an hour, we barely talk. If this neurosurgeon's prognosis should come true, then our son would proceed from the hospital to a chronic care facility. We'd never get to bring him home.

That night my husband and I lie in bed unable to fall asleep. In the dark, I can't make out the three gold-framed collages of baby pictures that hang above our headboard, but I know they're there. I try to picture Daniel growing older, living in some institution; still our son, but not a part of our daily lives. Will he even know who we are when we go to visit? Already Jonathan is reluctant to visit him. What will happen to the bond between my children? I can't imagine it. This may be worse than if he had died. With death comes a formal process for mourning; then life goes on. What about now? How are we supposed to conduct our lives? Turning to each other, we hug, desperate to hold on to whatever comfort we can. But even our touch feels painful, as if all of our skin cells were raw, exposed, and aching with grief. Releasing each other and turning away, I wonder if the social worker's prediction will come true. Will our marriage survive this tragedy?

The next afternoon after work, we meet Daniel's neurosurgeon in her office, a small room at the hospital overflowing with books beside an even smaller anteroom filled with half-packed boxes. When we're ushered in, she's seated at her desk, her fingers resting on the edge of a closed file. Dressed in a dark pantsuit with a bright blue blouse instead of green surgery garb, she could be a professor about to discuss a term paper with a failing student. Her voice is grave.

"My colleague told me he met with you yesterday. I'm also concerned that your son is showing spasticity in all four limbs. This isn't a good sign, as it suggests global damage."

"So, you agree with his predictions then," Joel says.

"No, despite these findings, I still believe that Daniel will be able to locomote and have self-help skills." A smile softens her serious demeanour and she glances at a picture frame of her own family that sits in the corner of her desk. "Even language is a possibility. If you'd like, I can have you meet another family whose son was in a coma three years ago. Now he's working on the family farm."

"But what about all that information we heard yesterday?"

"Maybe my colleague's approach is better," she muses. "Then

the worst-case scenario is anticipated and anything better would seem like a bonus. That's not my approach. I don't wish to give false hope, but I still believe in miracles, especially in the young."

As I start to feel the re-emergence of hope, she tempers her words, "Don't wait to grieve. You've definitely lost the son you had. I've tried to give you back a new son, but there are no guarantees."

We're getting our first lessons in the uncertainty of medical prediction and our core of trust in the experts is shaken. These two well-reputed doctors, each with years of experience, offer us such contrasting prognoses for our son. Which one should we believe? Daniel's surgeon, god-like, held his brain in her hands and wielded her trusty instruments. Yet even she admits that she can offer no assurance of the final outcome — the quality of the life she's saved.

Months later, I'll hear stories from other families of the inaccuracy of the early prognosis for their loved ones. Despite the predicted worst-case scenarios, many longed-for miracles come true.

But right now, we're numb, absorbing her message as we leave — *the Daniel we knew is gone forever.*

When I get home, Jonathan is sitting on the rug in the family room with the dog spread-eagled on her back between his legs. He rubs her belly, pressing his face into the thick white ruff of her neck as she nuzzles his face. When he lifts his head to say hello, I notice his furrowed brow.

"What's wrong?"

"I sit in class and try to listen, I really do. I keep thinking about Daniel though," he says.

I don't know what to say. He hasn't been to the hospital often, but he's been listening to our dinnertime discussions and understands the gravity of his brother's condition. Joel and I don't seem to talk about anything else these days. How can I tell Jonathan not to worry? Still, when he's in school, I'd like his focus to be there too. I make myself a mental note to call his guidance counsellor again tomorrow. Maybe she can help.

"What do you do at lunchtime?" I ask, wondering if he's also having adjustment problems in this new school setting.

"I know a lot of the kids already. But they keep complaining about their brothers or sisters. You know, like, 'He came into my room and took something,' or 'She wouldn't let me watch the TV show I wanted.'"

"Sounds typical. You guys used to do that all the time."

"Yeah, but I can't stand it. I wish Daniel were home to fight with me. I swear I wouldn't sneak into his room ever again."

"I wish he were here too. Do your classmates know about him?"

"No! And I don't want to tell them." He glares at me as if I might do so behind his back. I reassure him with a compassionate look. He sighs and continues, "Recess isn't bad. I just play basketball and don't have to think or talk at all."

I'd like to be able to ease Jonathan's pain. Describing the latest meeting with the neurosurgeon, I relay her best-case scenario.

"That's not good enough," he says.

I agree. Jonathan wants his brother to come home the way he was, but we can't turn back the clock and undo what's been done. We must focus on limiting the damage to the rest of the family. If only we knew how.

CHAPTER TWELVE

Finally, in his fourth week post-injury, Daniel is moved onto the neurological ward and placed in a semi-private room. In the bed closest to the window lies an older man who's had a stroke and has lost his ability to speak. We greet him politely. He doesn't turn his head; he just stares out the window. I follow his gaze through the slats in the blinds. There's nothing to see except another cinnamon-bricked building with more blind-covered windows. Joel carries the room's single chair over to Daniel's bed and we take turns sitting on it. We've been told that a coma can continue for weeks or even months. We can't get used to the slow pace, watching him just lie there, our son who was always a blur of motion.

Yellow, red, and green fragments whirl in my mind like a kaleidoscope. Red shorts and pudgy legs curved on the grass, fleshy folds of baby fat on tendrils of green. When he chortled, his whole body jiggled like my grandpa's belly. In his hand, the string of a yellow balloon bounced and bobbed, a reluctant sun lassoed and tugged across the sky.

I can picture the wide grin on his face on his third birthday when we presented his gift — a red plastic motorcycle big enough to ride on, covered with black and white decals. A twist of the handlebars, a motorized vroom, and then he was off, careening down the carpeted hallway. Outside, he'd race down the sidewalk, short legs pumping furiously; I'd have to jog alongside him just to keep up.

Now he just lies there, so still in bed, a rumpled T-shirt against crisp white sheets. There's a tube in his nose and one in his throat, an I.V. connected to his right arm. His cheeks are sunken and in his chin, the cleft is gouged as deeply as a furrow in freshly turned earth. Brown fuzz has started regrowing on his head, but doesn't yet cover the angry scar that runs from the top of his forehead to behind his left ear. The skin is pulled tautly where a bone flap was removed from his skull. We watch it vibrate, grey matter pulsing and bulging like a tennis ball above his left eyebrow.

His friends come to visit: Phil, Matt, Bijan, Benny, Jeremy, Jaimie, and Jared. My husband has trouble keeping their names straight. Most wear their hair long and are dressed in baggy shorts or torn jeans. Except for Phil, who comes alone, the guys advance down the hall in a group of three like an offensive line in hockey purposefully moving the puck forward. Their physical energy and booming male voices seem out of place in Daniel's half of the room.

"Hey man. How you doing? Feeling better today?"

"Dude, we missed you last night. Went out for wings, your favourite. Better get your ass out of here so you can come with us next time."

"Yeah, hockey season is about to start. We need you. Remember last year when you clunked Andrew on the head because he was more interested in showing off for Jodi than in chasing the puck?"

The nursing director pokes her head into the room, her voice like that of a schoolmarm. "Only two visitors at a time and could you *please* keep your voices down?"

"Yes, ma'am. Sorry." Respectfully, they lower their voices. One of the boys waits outside the room while the other two say goodbye to Daniel. As they exit the ward, their high-top sneakers flop open, unlaced and squeaking.

Joel attaches a poster to the ceiling so it hangs down right over Daniel's bed. Our son turns his head and looks up. Does he recognize it? This ski racer poster used to hang in his room beside his desk. His eyes blink, trying to focus. We're delighted at such a positive sign. The first of purposeful action.

I wonder what else my son sees? What he recognizes in this unfamiliar setting? Does he know who we are?

The next day, he turns his head towards the door when Phil walks in. With his sleeveless plaid shirt, khaki shorts, and sandals, Phil looks like he has just stepped out of a cabin at camp. Approaching the left side of the bed, he clasps Daniel's hand, his voice as gentle as a whispering wind.

"Hey, buddy. Looking good today. Want to hear about my job?"

He doesn't wait for an answer. "I'm working in the ski department of a sports store; you know, the big one on Yonge Street. They sent us out for a day of training to teach us about the different product lines. Wait 'til you see these new shaped skis they just brought in. You just think of turning and they do it."

"Mrs. Cohen?" he turns to me. "If Jonathan needs new equipment this year, send him to me and I'll get him a discount."

Already Daniel's eyes are drooping. His head lolls off the pillow. I stand up to straighten him out; Phil takes care of it before me.

As he turns to leave, he asks, "Mrs. Cohen, is there anything I can do to help? I've got flexible hours in my university courses this year so I can pop in. I'm not sure which days, though. It'll depend on my work schedule."

"That would be great, Phil. The physiotherapist just taught us how to do special exercises with Daniel to keep his joints limber. The next time you're in, I can show you them."

An hour later when his friend Jodi walks in, my son is still sleeping. She caresses the side of his face with her fingertips and readjusts the sheet over his shoulders.

"Shoot, I was hoping he'd be up. I just drove in from Montreal and I didn't even go home yet. My parents are going to kill me, but I had to see Daniel first. He's looking much better, isn't he?"

I nod my head.

"Like this fuzz. Wow, it's soft. I've already warned my folks that this is Daniel's weekend. I told them I'd be here all day tomorrow and Sunday, I'll be in early before I drive back."

"Jodi, visiting hours don't even start until eleven in the morning."

"Don't worry. The nurses will let me in. I'm so quiet, they won't even know I'm here."

Suddenly looking very tired, she leans on the bars of his bed.

"Why don't you go home now and come back later? His nurse has given him a shot of codeine and he'll probably sleep for a while."

"No, I'll just stay here and rest a bit."

"Well then, take my chair. I'll go for a short walk."

Outside on the hospital steps, I pause to take a deep breath, filling my lungs with fresh air. Alyssa will be here tonight, home for the weekend, and I can't wait. Her visits always buoy us up. Like Jodi, who speaks of the soft brown fuzz covering my son's head, not the ugly scar, my daughter projects the optimism of youth. Daniel's friends all do. Perhaps they haven't grasped the implications of the uncertain outcome. More likely, they can't allow themselves to consider that the Daniel they know won't ever return. I set off and walk briskly around the perimeter of the hospital complex, passing grey monolithic buildings that skirt the parking lot.

When I return, Jodi is asleep, curled up like a lithe cat, her legs tugged under her and her blond ponytail streaming over her right shoulder.

Two days later, the nursing director approaches us. Today her voice is calm and friendly. "Your son gets so many visitors I decided it would be better if he were in a private room. That way his current roommate can get more rest. A room will be available tomorrow.

Is this all right with you?" We're delighted.

We hang up pictures and posters, trying to bring a sense of Daniel's own space into the sterile hospital room. His blue and gold hockey shirt and a photo of last year's team with the guys all clowning around and mugging for the camera. A picture from summer camp of the water-ski staff. He was so proud to be one of the elite — hugging his slalom ski, his most prized possession.

Daniel had paid for his ski, a Kidder Red Line, with his own money, saved from birthday gifts and part-time work at the take-out counter of a local restaurant. The ski had a double boot instead of the usual open back pocket, and was sized so tightly he had to grease his feet to slip them in. He would just whiz through the slalom course, his shoulders almost skimming the water's surface, a huge spray streaming out behind him as proudly as a peacock's tail.

Now the only stream is yellow, dripping from a catheter into a bag. I watch as his nurse, Lynn, removes the full bag and exchanges it for an empty one. Lynn's short hair bobs as she props him on one side, balancing him in place with extra pillows. Whipping the soiled linens from the left half of the bed, she quickly replaces them with fresh sheets. Then she flips him over and after rearranging the pillows, finishes the task, smoothing the sheets with her palm.

"There you go, sir. Nice fresh linens. How does that feel?" Smiling at him, she changes the protein bag on his feeding tube and adjusts the flow.

"Oh, wow, a new poster. The Tragically Hip, your favourite group. Who brought it? Was it Jodi? I saw her in here a few days ago."

Lynn walks over to the windowsill and picking up the journal, reads yesterday's entry.

"Boy, did you ever have a lot of visitors last night. No wonder you're tired. Better rest up. Jennifer is going to be in soon to work with you."

The physiotherapist, Jennifer, is a slim young woman with a long blond braid that bounces down her back. She cranks up the bed and shifts Daniel to the right side of it. Working behind him, she manoeuvres him into a seated position. His head wobbles and his chin starts to fall forward onto his chest. Jennifer's muscles are taut as she pulls him back against her to straighten him out.

"C'mon, you can do this. Look at that picture of you and Phil on the wall over there."

His head rises slightly.

"You've got to sit before you can stand." She touches his chin and guides it higher. "A little bit more. That's it. Good work."

My son is now seated almost upright and balanced within the physiotherapist's outstretched arms. When he's lying back in bed, propped on his side again with pillows, Jennifer turns to me. I'm sitting on the edge of my chair, my breath ragged as if I too had just finished a strenuous workout.

"I got a message from your husband asking if he could try this sitting exercise. Please tell him, not yet. I'll let him know when Daniel's more stable. In the meantime, keep working on those passive range-of-motion exercises. They really help."

CHAPTER THIRTEEN

On Thursday afternoons, there's a trauma support group for the families of patients on the neurological ward. A month has now passed since Daniel was admitted to the hospital and it's the first meeting I'm attending. My mother comes with me. At 3:00 p.m. on the dot, we enter a room that has hospital-issue furniture: orange vinyl chairs that are grouped in a circle, a plain wooden table covered with files, and beige walls with nothing but medical diagrams for decoration. The two leaders, women in their thirties, greet us warmly, inviting us to sit down and help ourselves to coffee and cookies that are displayed on a tray in the centre of the circle.

My mother sits on the edge of her chair and whispers, "Aren't any others coming?"

There are eight empty chairs around us.

"How can we help you?" one leader asks.

I'm not sure what to say. "Can you tell me how long a coma lasts?"

From the wooden table behind her, she reaches for a plastic model of the brain and holds it aloft. Each lobe is shaded with a different primary colour. The brain separates like a child's puzzle. She takes it apart and starts explaining the functions of the different parts of the brain.

"The brain stem, the base of the brain, is the site for autonomic nervous functions. It's like a reptilian brain, controlling sleep, temperature control, breathing, and the like."

Carefully reconstructing the pieces as she talks, she works her way to the left frontal hemisphere, demonstrating for us the area where my son sustained the most damage to his brain.

"The left side of the brain controls the right side of the body. That's why you see the hemiparesis" — I know she means weakness — "on his right side. This section also houses the language area of the brain."

We're getting a lesson in basic brain anatomy, but she still hasn't answered my question. I ask again. "How long does a coma last?"

"Each individual is different. There are no set time frames, but based on what you've told me, his coma appears to be lightening."

The other leader asks, "Tell us how you're doing."

"I wish there was more I could do to help," my mother says.

"You're here with your daughter. That's important."

I reach over, pat my mother's arm, and smile at her. "We're all trying to support one another; we're just not sure what to do. Our other kids are back in school and my husband and I still go to work. The rest of the time, we're here in the hospital with Daniel."

"That's great," she tells us.

Great? We're going through the motions of normal life. Jonathan says little. One of us tries to be at home with him in the evenings as we take turns visiting Daniel, but I don't expect that we're much company and our youngest often retreats to his bedroom or to the basement to watch television.

Great? I feel overwhelmed by sadness. Family and friends are aching along with us and whenever Ellen drops in, I cry. I wonder if like a hurt animal, I should retreat to be alone with my pain. There's anger in me too, although it doesn't bubble to the surface like Joel's. In the safety of our bedroom, he curses Daniel's friend for his stupid driving and shouts his rage at our son for not listening and following the care we taught him, for not wearing his seatbelt, for throwing his life away.

Great? We're trying to hold our lives together while mourning the loss of our son — our son who is still alive.

When my mother and I leave the meeting room, the coffee and cookies remain untouched.

October 3, 1993

Dear Family and Friends,

6:30 a.m. I can't sleep. My stomach is in knots. Five weeks ago at this time, my family was whole. We were all at the cottage — Daniel with his friends — but by the end of that day, our lives were turned upside down, and like Humpty Dumpty, "couldn't be put together again." Other clichés keep spinning through my head: "You can't turn the clock back." "You have to take one day at a time."

You all know about his injury, so I won't go over it again. At the moment, Daniel is still considered to be in a coma, although it is lightening. We have been keeping a journal in his room so that visitors can write in their observations of his state and actions. The journal serves several purposes. It enables us to keep track of his progress and to mark the changes that occur. The staff who work with Daniel can check to see what he's doing for family and friends because patients will often respond more with familiar people than with professionals. In addition, it will serve as a record for Daniel who may some day want to know what occurred during this time frame.

Daniel is becoming more aware of his surroundings and has started responding more consistently. When he is responsive he will follow simple commands such as, "Close your eyes, open your hand, lift your leg." He is interested in the pictures and posters we have hung around the room and will turn his head to see them. If a picture is held in front of him, he will track it with his eyes. One morning, Daniel tracked the arrival of people in his room, turning his head whenever someone new walked in. While this behaviour is still not consistent, these signs are positive and indicate movement in the right direction.

At times you feel Daniel is looking directly at you and you wonder how much he really understands. At other times, his gaze is vacant and he looks "spacey," a name we used to call him when he would be engrossed in a TV show or SEGA game and oblivious to anything else.

The physiotherapist showed me, Sue, and Ellen (a close friend) how to do passive range-of-motion with Daniel. This involves exercising the joints in his shoulders, elbows, wrists, hips, and knees so they don't lose their flexibility. Ellen is going to train a few other friends also who will each visit once a week to help out. The physiotherapist will continue to work with Daniel as well. When possible, she likes to have his position changed by moving him to a chair or to a tilt table. The latter is a contraption that Daniel gets strapped to that is then tilted in an upright position so it simulates standing.

Last Wednesday, the fracture clinic started the first of a series of casts on Daniel's feet and right arm. This procedure is meant to prevent tendons from shortening. Daniel has not been moving his right arm or leg on his own, although his left arm and leg are moving vigorously. It amazes me how high he can lift his leg and he swings it with such force that you have to be careful not to be hit by the cast.

The occupational therapist, Alison, visits Daniel twice a day on the three days that she's in. Alison has met with us on several occasions and manages to convey a sense of hope. She has given us suggestions for providing Daniel with stimulation without overloading him. She's pleased that he is having so many visitors, for she feels that family and friends can provide that special "extra" that can't be measured directly in the rehabilitation process.

Daniel's friends have been terrific. Several of his friends call and even visit Jonathan so he doesn't feel left out. Daniel has five or six close friends who visit regularly, but there are more than twenty friends who keep dropping in. One friend, Jodi, is particularly special. She is away at university in Montreal this year, but has been coming home for the holidays. When she's in town she spends hours at the hospital with Daniel. She has such optimism that it's contagious. We know that most of these teenagers will not be able to sustain this level of commitment, but we certainly appreciate it for now.

Joel and I are both back at work physically, if not mentally. This is the time of our lives to be obsessed with Daniel. We're holding up as best we can. Joel and I cannot believe the outpouring of love and support that we are receiving. The phone lines across Canada and the U.S. and to Israel don't stop ringing. I'm so glad that there's an efficient grapevine.

Jonathan provides the noise and laughter that we've come to expect in our household. He's going through a growth spurt and enjoys standing right in front of me, looking over my head, and asking "Where's Mom?" He has started a new school this year, where he's in grade nine. He knew many kids already and has made new friends also. He's finding the adjustment difficult as his concentration is affected by what's going on with Daniel. Jonathan is riding the emotional roller coaster with us, but is insulated somewhat by social activities. Hockey starts for him this week, which should provide some fun.

Alyssa had trouble forcing herself to return to university, as she felt she was needed here. She was accepted into an intensive two-year program — honours business administration. We convinced her to go, and she is now so involved that she has little time to think. She is either in class, preparing for the next class on her own or with her study group, or sleeping. How she fits in the time for swimming and socializing is beyond me. She and her roommates have arranged for a Toronto phone number so they pay a flat rate per month instead of long distance rates to call home. We speak to her regularly and she has been coming home for the holidays. We expect she'll be back every second or third weekend. We're lucky London is only a two-hour drive from Toronto (in non-rush hour traffic, of course).

We hope you're being kept informed through the proper channels. We'll try to update everyone when we can. If prayers and hope work, Daniel should be on his way to recovery. We're waiting for a miracle!

With love,
Lainie

Part Two

"Joel, you'd better pick up the phone. It's Alyssa. She says she wants to come home tonight and it sounds like she won't take no for an answer."

"Hi, cutie," he says. "What's up?"

There's a brief pause. I can picture our daughter girding herself for battle, her arms crossed against her chest, steeling her voice with determination like a lawyer about to give her final summation speech to a jury. I know she's upset about staying in London this weekend. We'd talked her into it, wanting to give her a chance to catch up on her studies, but it seems like our plans have backfired. She says she feels left out and must see for herself what's happening.

There's not much happening. Daniel's progress is slow, so much slower than we had anticipated, and our lives revolve around visits to the hospital. Sometimes Joel and I go together. More often, we go alone, so one of us can be home with Jonathan.

My car seems to have taken on a life on its own, insulating me from the world outside as it heads to the hospital down Bayview Avenue, passing the plaza, hockey arena, film centre, private boys' school, the large homes with their gracious lawns. It stops, almost of its own accord, for me to reach for a parking ticket, and then spirals slowly down the ramp to the first available parking spot. I get out and walk, the too-familiar walk through the garage and up the stone steps of Building C, through the wood-panelled lobby decorated with portraits of former chairmen of the hospital, to the elevator where I wait to be transported to the fifth floor.

I'm filled with a strange mixture of trepidation and excitement each time I enter Daniel's room. Will he be awake this visit? Will he be responsive? I scan the journal entries that his visitors write, eagerly searching for signs of improvement. Yesterday, my sister-in-law Roz noted that Daniel's eyes followed the sound of her voice and he blinked when my nephew Brian asked if Daniel knew who he was. Was the blink just a reflex? We've been trying to teach him to blink as a signal for yes. Sometimes, though, it's hard to determine what's intentional behaviour, as Daniel's responses are often delayed.

When Alyssa arrives late that night, Joel and I are relieved to see her safely home. We stand in the front hall hugging her, an uneven tripod on the shiny marble floor, the curved oak banister on the stairway steadily reflected in the mirrored doors.

"Do you want anything to eat?" I ask.

Wearily, she shakes her head.

"Then, you'd better get to sleep."

Joel carries her knapsack upstairs and she follows, passing by Jonathan's closed door and Daniel's open one right next to hers. When she turns on the light, her room springs to life with her floral quilt of white, purple, and green, her white eyelet pillows, billowy curtains, and deep purple carpet like lush velvet moss. On shelves and atop bureaus sprout a wild garden of photos and files, books and knick-knacks in porcelain and brass. There's a scent here too — fresh body lotion and raspberry candles in heart-shaped glass bowls.

She flops on her bed. When I bend to kiss her good night, her long hair brushes my cheek, and I'm comforted by her feel.

At dinnertime the next day, four of us sit around the table together. Jonathan is talkative for a change. Spearing pasta noodles quickly, he tells us how surprised he was when Alyssa picked him up from school.

"She even gave my friend a lift home before we went to visit Daniel."

Joel and I smile at him and try to avoid looking at the empty chair between us.

After dinner, I join Alyssa for her third visit that day to the hospital. We've been trying to follow the speech therapist's suggestion to have Daniel follow one-step commands. Alyssa picks up Daniel's old teddy bear and holds it towards him. As a toddler, he slept on Teddy instead of a pillow, his wayward brown locks nestled into fuzzy blue fur. Now Teddy's stuffing is flattened, the freckles on its nose have disappeared, and there's only a hint of colour left in the formerly red lips. Daniel reaches past the bear and tries to take hold of his sister's hand instead. Is he again confused and not able to follow her simple direction? Then he lifts his arm and places it on her back. Alyssa's green-grey eyes glisten.

"Daniel, that feels great. I love when you hug me."

I watch in amazement thinking: This is better than just turning his head to look at a ski poster. That doctor was wrong. Daniel does know us.

I move to the left side of the bed and he "hugs" me too. I can't believe how good it feels. It's taken such effort to get a hug from my son in recent years. His favourite way before his injury was to put both arms around me like a big brown bear, then gently pat me on the back.

"Nice little Mom," he'd say.

Now his lips move as if he's trying to say something. I listen hard, but no sound comes out.

One afternoon when I visit, I take out a letter that's just arrived from his friend, Rachel, who's spending the year studying in Switzerland. Her letter is long and chatty, mostly about her classes, wine festivals, and some sightseeing trips. My son's eyes begin to droop and I'm about to put away the letter when suddenly they pop open. I've just read her reminiscence of the late evening canoe rides they took together at camp, the moon shining on the docks and the calm water, how Daniel would listen to her talking about her campers and tell her about the kids he had taken water-skiing that day. He seems much more alert, so interested now. Does he really process this information differently? Can he remember the events she writes about?

There's a soft knock on the door and a young man nervously pokes his head into the room. He looks the same as when I last saw him, sitting in the driver's seat that late August day as he drove Daniel away from the cottage. Was it just five weeks ago? His straight black hair still brushes below his eyebrows and he sweeps his hand up to remove his bangs from his eyes.

"May I come in?" John asks. "Matt and Jaimie spoke to Mr. Cohen. He told them I could visit."

Folding Rachel's letter, I tuck it into the night table by my son's bed. Uncomfortably, I turn and face the visitor.

"Sure, John," I say with forced politeness. "How are you?"

"Well, I have to wear this back brace for another few weeks, but I'm okay. How's Daniel?"

"Coming along, we hope."

"Yeah, I heard. The guys have been keeping me up-to-date."

He steps gingerly to the other side of the bed. My eyes skitter around him. I can barely bring myself to look at him. Why is he standing here talking to me while my son lies silently in a hospital bed? Inwardly I scream it's not fair.

We've already spoken to the police officer who shared the news of Daniel's injury with Alyssa, and to several other police investigators as well. We had little to tell them. Everything seemed fine when the boys left our cottage around 5:00 p.m. that afternoon. When the police examined the remains of the car, they found no evidence of alcohol or drugs to suggest impaired driving ability. The road conditions were also ideal that day — warm, dry, clear visibility. From what they could gather, traffic had been unusually slow on the main highway and the boys had turned off to take an alternate route. It's unclear what happened next, but based on reports from other drivers, the police are surmising that the car crash was a result of driver error involving excessive speed.

Excessive speed. Failure to merge. Right tires skidding on the shoulder, then loss of control. Metal defying gravity. My son's blood seeping into the grass.

Taken aback by the vividness of these images, I find myself trembling. I look at John, standing awkwardly near his friend's bed. Is he picturing the same scene? Seeing himself and Daniel speeding along on that bright summer day and wishing that it had turned out differently?

Must get out of here, I tell myself. Pull myself back together.

"I'll leave you alone," I say. "I've been meaning to check out the office of the Brain Injury Association. It's somewhere in this hospital."

"Sure, Mrs. Cohen. Take your time. I'll be here and . . . thanks."

I hesitate near the open doorway. The lone occupant in the office, who is talking on the phone, beckons me in. The small room is crammed with books, videos, binders, and a bulletin board with yellow Post-it notes, giving it a sense of overwhelming chaos. What am I doing here? The woman looks too busy to be of any help. She has short grey hair and a bustling manner that reminds me of the nurses on the ward. Holding up a finger to indicate she'll be with me in a moment, she waves me to the only other chair in the room — one that's covered with magazines and papers. Seamlessly, she continues her conversation, taking notes as she listens. Still shaken from my encounter with John, I remove the magazines and cautiously balance them near the edge of her desk. Perching uneasily on the chair, I wait.

When she hangs up the phone, she turns to greet me. "Hi, I'm Esther, the information officer. How can I help you?"

"My son's in this hospital. He's been here for five weeks. A severe brain injury." I speak in staccato blurts like the toot, toot, toot of a train whistle as it passes a level crossing, warning of danger, and I burst into tears.

Esther reaches for a Kleenex box and hands it to me.

"Oh, I know just what you're going through." Her hand gently touches mine and her eyes share her story before her words can express it. "My son had a severe brain injury too, nine years ago."

"I'm so scared. I don't know what's going to happen to him."

Esther listens. I tell her what's happened. She asks me some questions and I tell her some more. Somehow, I get a sense of comfort pouring out my fears to her. There's no pooh-poohing, telling me not to worry, that everything will be okay. Just listening from someone who has been there herself and truly understands.

"I'm going to give you some material to read," she tells me. "Just give me a minute and I'll look for the articles I think you'll find helpful. While I'm making copies, you're welcome to look through our library for any books or videos you might want. There are a few I'd like to recommend."

As I leave the office, I realize that I haven't much time to read the material Esther's given me. Only eight days now before my psychology exam and everywhere I go, I carry one of the study guides and a deck of index cards with me. Fluorescent pink and yellow lines highlight the important points I'm trying to learn. Joel understands my fixation and is pleased I have something else to focus on other than Daniel. I'm not sure how Jonathan feels. His feelings and thoughts seem bottled up tightly inside him. Although I try to spend time with him, he says little to me, little to anyone.

The next morning before I leave for work, I take the first of eight practice tests, thinking the multiple-choice format should be easy. The results are demoralizing. I'm totally confused by the statistical concept of false positives and negatives in testing, and I've botched all those questions.

Alyssa had explained the concept to me in August, her coursework in statistics more recent than mine, which came during the sixties at McGill University. Sitting together at the picnic table on the deck of our cottage, she wrote out examples for me on a pad of lined yellow paper. I'd been a teacher myself — my first career — and I remember thinking she would make a fine educator too, her explanation so clear and concise that in less than an hour, I had grasped it. It seemed so obvious then. Now I wish I could recall what she taught me, but the information seems to slide from my memory as readily as an egg from a Teflon pan.

Maybe my mother is right after all. She's worried I'm pushing myself too hard. Perhaps I should defer the exam until it's given again next April.

That afternoon I'm back at the hospital, still thinking of testing and tests.

"Hi, Daniel," I call cheerily when I enter his room, pleased that he's awake.

He doesn't turn his head towards me. His eyes flit about the room — the posters, the photos, the stacked games on the window ledge — not alighting on anything for long. I approach his bed. It's as if I'm not there. He seems to look right through me.

Damn, I hate this. The hopeful stage of hugs is gone. He's been non-responsive for days now. The nurses say it's just a phase, but it feels like a regression to me.

I pick up a ski magazine and start to flip through it. "Can you point to the skier? See the one in the red jacket."

My son lifts his left hand and vigorously rubs his ear.

I try a few more activities. Testing, testing . . . but Daniel doesn't follow any of my instructions and drifts off to sleep.

Sitting in the chair near the window, I find myself clutching the arms of the chair. Suddenly I can see myself as I was ten years ago standing at a swimming pool, clenching the edge with my toes, my arms raised above my head, ready to dive. I remember how cold the water felt, but I didn't give myself a chance to do a gradual warm-up. There were just two weeks left until the qualification class for the bronze medallion test and I was having trouble increasing my speed to complete twenty laps within fourteen minutes.

Bend your elbow, extend your hand forward, keep your fingers cupped. Pull the water. It was as if the instructor's voice were right in my ear, even though I was practising alone that night. My palms cupped the liquid and forced it back. *Don't forget your legs. Keep kicking. That's it. Now, turn and breathe.* At the end of the pool, I neatly executed a jackknife turn underwater. My arms moved like pistons, up and over, up and over again. Counting off the required twelve lengths of front crawl, I switched to four laps of breaststroke and finally flipped over onto my back for the last four lengths of legs only. By now, my legs felt like rubber, detached somehow from the rest of me, my feet paddling like an upside-down duck. I wished that I too had webbing between my toes to propel me faster. When finished, I removed my goggles and gazed at the clock. Damn, still fifteen seconds over the allotted time.

The night of the swim test, we all lined up at the side of the pool. Aside from one fellow who also appeared to be in his mid-thirties, the rest were self-conscious teenagers. The girls stood around giggling, flipping the hair out of their eyes; the boys leaned against the wall, arms crossed in macho fashion over their bare chests. At fifteen-second intervals, we were directed to dive into the pool and begin swimming our laps. There were four of us in each lane, and the other swimmers quickly overtook me.

Focus. Don't think of them. You can do this, I told myself. And somehow I did.

The next morning at breakfast, when I displayed my bronze medallion award, a small copper-coloured disk, Alyssa said, "Too bad you didn't get a badge like my Red Cross green award that you could sew on your bathing suit."

I just nodded and tucked the small medallion into my pant pocket. Throughout the day, my fingers rubbed it like a magical talisman.

From my briefcase, I remove the study guide I began reviewing this morning. I open it on my lap and begin to read. Only eight more days until the test. There's still a lot of information to cover.

Beside me, Daniel sleeps.

CHAPTER FIFTEEN

Week six: I sit in the corner of his room, watching my son, his chest rising and falling in a steady rhythm. Daniel's feeding tube makes an irregular click; the liquid drips, gathering at a bottle-neck before whooshing through the tube. My seat is right under the window, and from my fifth-floor vantage point, I can look out at the covered windows of the adjoining hospital wing, and at a shingled roof if I crane my head a little. There are no trees or other greenery to break the monotony of the brown bricks and black shingles, no people to see, no cars to watch. Pulling out a file from my briefcase, I try to concentrate on my work while I wait for my son to awaken.

The sheets rustle as his left arm and leg begin to stretch. Soon his eyes will open and we'll begin our work together. I start with physical stretching exercises, the passive range-of-motion activities that the physiotherapist taught us to keep his right side mobile. He has some movement in his right shoulder joint, but he can't move his right leg at all on his own. Lifting his leg, I press his knee into his chest and then rotate it sideways. How heavy his leg feels in my arms. He just lies there, oblivious to my actions. After ten repetitions, I turn my attention to his arm, following the prescribed routine. When I stretch his arm overhead, he grimaces and I count off the repetitions like a trainer in a gym, "And five, and six . . . only four more to go. That's it. Keep working. Good."

Now comes the stimulation program. I rub him with various textures: silk, cotton, corduroy, even a piece of light sandpaper. From smooth to rough, rough to smooth, I name each texture as I touch his cheek and bare chest, my fingers lingering against his warm skin, in the curls of dark hair under the scar in his throat. What can he feel? A wisp of cotton on the back of his hand? The scratch of sandpaper on the sole of his foot? There's no change in his eyes, no movement in his body.

I crank up the bed so he's now semi-reclining, then reach for the box of spice jars on the windowsill, wafting one at a time under his nostrils. Nose-crinkling ammonia contrasts with the sweet smell of cinnamon. The latter reminds me of one of his favourite desserts — apple crisp. If I didn't hide it, a big chunk would be gone before supper was served. I remember placing little Post-it notes on apple cakes before Friday night dinners, "Don't even think of eating this. Guests coming." How long ago it seems.

Picking up a package of Scratch 'n' Sniff stickers, I scratch pictures of peppermint, pineapples, pickles, and pizza, holding them under his nose. Am I teasing him with these tantalizing smells of food? He's just had his feeding tube changed from his nose to his stomach and isn't permitted to eat anything by mouth. His nose wrinkles, but of course, he says nothing. He's still not able to talk.

Although there's so much more I want to do, he's already beginning to tire. Perhaps later I'll show him photos from our family album or pictures from magazines he used to enjoy, *Sports Illustrated* and *Ski Canada*. He's just learning how to point and is still inconsistent in following directions, but we keep working on these activities. Maybe tomorrow . . .

Sometimes while Daniel sleeps, I get restless and pace around the ward, where the halls form a large U-shape with the busy nursing station in the centre. I wish that I could stroll through a leafy green promenade or a boardwalk by the sea with the smell of fresh ocean breezes. Instead, there's a pervasive hospital smell — antiseptic solutions and soiled linens. At mealtimes, the food in covered trays has no smell at all, no enticing aroma from rubbery sandwiches, plastic eggs, and watery coffee. I walk past rooms that are usually so quiet. Most house older long-term patients who've had strokes and are waiting to be moved into nursing homes. In some, the hustle and bustle of visitors, fresh flowers, and balloons on a bureau top signal a recent arrival. Glancing in, I'm aware of my intrusion on others' privacy, and walk quickly by those open doorways.

Other times I slow down to nod and smile at patients sitting in the hall.

My favourite is an older, silver-haired gentleman. He looks

dapper with his moustache trimmed evenly, his cheeks clean-shaven, and his shirt collar buttoned. Beside his wheelchair, his wife constantly sits, patting or resting her hand on his, as if they were young sweethearts. She's always dressed in matching sweaters and skirts, with a bright scarf or pin that sparkles in the fluorescent light. And she always smiles, a brave grin that flickers when her head is turned away from her husband.

The quiet of the hallway is sometimes disrupted by the agitated voices of visitors on the payphone just outside the lounge, and of course, by Charlene. Much younger than most of the patients on the ward, she always positions her wheelchair right beside the nursing station, where she sits, sucking on her stringy straw-coloured hair, and beseeching every staff member who passes, "Going for a smoke? Will you take me?"

When I walk by, she reaches for my sleeve, "Hey Miss, take me downstairs?"

A nurse's voice pipes up from behind the counter, "Give it a rest, Charlene. The attendants aren't here right now. You'll have to wait for the breaks to be finished. We'll let you know."

Occasionally, there's an unexpected drama, like the day a truck driver stomped down the hall, dangling his jacket from one hand and pulling his girlfriend in tow with the other.

"The doctors are crazy here, not me. I don't need no tests. I didn't have no brain injury. I didn't even have no accident like they say. They're nuts. I'm outta here," he bellowed.

His girlfriend whimpered, trying to reason with him, trying to keep up with him. I never saw them again.

One evening, I'm surprised to hear the wail of a child. Rushing out of Daniel's room, I see a young woman leaning on the wall a few doors away. She's carrying an infant in one arm and is bending to hug her three- or four-year-old daughter, whose face is buried against her mother's legs.

"It's okay, sweetie. Daddy looks a little funny and can't talk to you right now, but he's going to be just fine."

The young woman becomes a daily visitor. We exchange stories. When a transport truck hit her husband's car, he sustained a severe brain injury not unlike my son's. We compare notes and I offer to share what I've learned. She isn't ready to hear it yet. She still needs to believe that life will progress like a movie or television program with an instant cure to coma.

"My Kevin will be just fine, you'll see. Your Daniel will, too."

Some days I believe her. Other days I'm not so sure.

CHAPTER SIXTEEN

When my husband came home from the hospital yesterday, he was more animated than I've seen him in ages. Seven weeks now since Daniel's injury, and Joel is beaming.

"I think Daniel can read," Joel said.

"What are you talking about?"

"I took a piece of cardboard and a purple marker and wrote his name. He looked at it and seemed to squint. I outlined each letter and coloured them all in, forming thick block print. He stared at it and blinked his eyes. We've got to try this again."

Today, when I arrive at the hospital after work, my son is sitting in the hallway outside his room in a geri chair — a reclining chair — with his feeding tube attached to a pole just behind him. The chair is massive, an expanse of blue vinyl on wheels, with a tray over his lap that helps to position him in place and hold him semi-upright. Daniel's eyes appear bright. Placing a chair beside him, I pull out a deck of homemade word cards with names of family members and friends that Joel and I made last night.

"Does this say 'Joel'?" I ask, holding up a card in front of him.

He blinks his eyes once, his signal for "yes."

Amazed, I hold up the same card again. "Does this say Alyssa?" This time he doesn't blink.

Is this a fluke or can he really read? We go through a few cards accurately before he turns his head away and doesn't respond at all.

Still, I'm encouraged, and arrange to meet with the speech pathologist. Later that afternoon, she taps briskly on the door to Daniel's room. Not wishing to disturb my sleeping son, I rise from my chair and meet her in the hallway. She carries her briefcase, instead of setting it down on the floor, appearing impatient to move on to something else. She's obviously very busy. I avoid any small talk and plunge right into my question.

"Could we use an alternative form of communication with Daniel?" I ask. "Perhaps some non-verbal form of pictographs would work."

"Until he shows consistency in following simple one-step commands, there's little point in working on other aspects of language," she says.

"But he seems to respond better to visual stimuli than to auditory. How do we know that progress will be linear?"

"I've had years of experience working with patients with brain injury," she replies, ending the interview.

Her briefcase swings by her side as she walks down the hall, her head held high and confident. I'm filled with a sudden dislike of the woman. How well does she even know our son? She seems more concerned with the status of his swallowing than anything else.

That evening when I relate the conversation to Joel, he too becomes angry.

"The experts don't know it all," he says, "even if they think they do. Find out what you need and we'll use it together."

I phone my close friend Barb, a speech pathologist, feeling lucky to have this connection. I wonder what other families do without the support of such friends. Perhaps, like the wife of the young man who's in the room down the hall from Daniel, they wait patiently for events to unfold, believing that the hospital staff is doing all that's needed, all that can be done. Perhaps their faith is greater or maybe they're just overwhelmed by the catastrophic events that have felled their loved one. Joel and I can't function that way. We see how stretched the medical resources are. Even when staff members are willing to help, they're pressed for time and can't do enough. Besides, we need to be doing something — something that might speed this process along — whatever it takes to help our son.

Barb refers me to a colleague who works in another hospital setting. This woman listens attentively, questioning what's been working and what hasn't. I answer honestly, trying to paint a realistic picture of Daniel's difficulty in sustaining attention and his lack of consistency. I'm relieved when she agrees that my ideas are worth trying. She tells me about the Augmentative Communication Centre where support is given to school-age children and adolescents who have problems with verbal communication.

"There's a long waiting list for service, but I know someone who works there. Give her my name and I'm sure she'll be able to give you some guidance if you're willing to do this yourself."

The clinician shows me samples of booklets made for other non-verbal clients. The range is large — a single folded page with family photos, an album of cut-out magazine pictures, a personal dictionary filled with stick-figure symbols — all labelled with words and some with sentences. A few booklets have rings to hang from a wheelchair. Others are thin and cardboard-backed to fit snugly in a pocket. I leave with my head swimming with possibilities.

On the way home, I stop at a camera store to buy a photo album with adhesive pages. The bright coral binding attracts me, and I pick an album whose cover has a photograph of a mallard duck paddling in clear blue water. That night, I begin working on a communication binder. Joel joins me, and together we brainstorm what to include: line drawings of personal care items and simple instructions about turning the light on and off and raising and lowering the bed. We choose large thick type as we don't know how clear Daniel's eyesight is; the occupational therapist suspects that he might be suffering from double vision.

The first page has two sentences, "I have to pee. I need a bedpan," and three pictures — a urinal, a bedpan, and a stick figure with wet pants. We hope we can help Daniel regain continence if he can express his needs using the binder. Optimistically, I include a list of games my son likes to play. Maybe we can get his friends to use this binder and play games with him when they come to visit.

The occupational therapist gives me a list of suggestions to share with visitors, so I post a sheet of instructions on the door to Daniel's hospital room.

TIPS FOR VISITORS

1. Identify yourself: "Hi, Daniel. It's _____."
2. Place yourself in his line of vision if necessary to get eye contact.
3. If the radio or TV is on, turn it off during your visit.
4. Tell Daniel when you are going to touch him.
5. If there is more than one of you, have only one person talk at a time.
6. Talk to him about familiar events, places, and people. Talk about experiences you have shared.
7. Praise him if he responds to you.
8. Tell him that he is getting better and you are going to help him.
9. Please note in the diary your name, the time of your visit, and what you observed. We use this information to keep track of when Daniel is most responsive and to help with memory training.

Thank you for visiting. We hope you'll come again soon.

The number of visitors Daniel has amazes the nursing staff, and us as well. Matt and his girlfriend Caroline, Jaimie, Laurel, Bijan, and

Phil all drop in several times a week. Jodi comes by whenever she's in town, and John, the driver of the car, visits almost every day. John isn't attending classes this semester; he plans to start again in January. When he visits, I don't run out of the room anymore. I still feel somewhat unsettled, but I've seen the way my son's face lights up when he recognizes his friend.

Other friends surface unexpectedly like clowns springing out of a tiny circus car and sign their names in the journal we keep on the windowsill. There are so many, I can't imagine where they all come from. I meet Daniel's former girlfriends and learn who has his missing sweatshirt, the one he claimed he'd lost in camp. And I hear stories about my son, this young man we thought we knew. Some guys talk of skipping class with him to grab breakfast at some greasy diner. Others tell tales of getting drunk and getting high. What surprises me most is how my son — who could be so stingy with words at home — was so articulate in his English class, readily offering opinions on texts that I never knew he'd read. I long to hear his voice again.

The nursing director drops in one day while my friend, Ellen, is training a volunteer to perform the passive range-of-motion exercises that the physiotherapist taught us.

"Boy, I wish we could get this support for all our patients," she says. "With the cutbacks to health care, my nurses don't have the time to do everything that's needed."

We're so lucky. Four of my friends and my sister-in-law Sue each take a turn during the week to do these exercises with Daniel. Phil joins in each time he comes. Other friends and family members visit too, keeping us company in the evenings and on weekends. Some visitors seem to have a natural knack and manage to carry on a relaxed conversation with Daniel. Others are nervous, unsure what to say, so uncomfortable with the silence that greets their remarks that they talk at the rate of a mile-a-minute. One fellow keeps up a running monologue for ten minutes straight and looks drained by the time he leaves, exhausting me, too, just by listening.

My son is sleeping the day that Ellen arrives with her son, Robert. Robert's glossy red hair hangs in curls below his shoulders and his freckled face smiles as I get up from the chair to hug him. I know Robert well. He and Daniel were best friends for years, from the time they travelled to the same nursery school each morning. Even then, Robert was the talker, chattering non-stop; my son was the quieter sidekick. They played on the same competitive hockey teams, practically lived in each other's homes, and spent time together at our cottage. After we moved to a new neighbourhood when Daniel was thirteen, they drifted apart, each mixing with new friends, but today that distance fades.

Robert takes one look at his friend, bald again following recent surgery to replace his bone flap, and collapses in the chair beneath the window. His knees curl up to his chin and his chest heaves with sobs. I watch, saddened, as Ellen gently leads her son from the room.

SECOND NEWSLETTER

October 27, 1993
Dear Family and Friends,

Changes have occurred since the last time I wrote. Daniel had his trach removed on Saturday, October 9. The following Wednesday, when Joel was visiting and told him that it was time for him to leave, Daniel shook his head no. He did the same thing later when two friends were leaving. He also put his hand on his friend's arm and made a groaning sound as if to say "no."

On Friday, October 15, he had the nasogastric tube removed from his nose. He had found it quite irritating and kept trying to pull it out, succeeding so many times that he was having nosebleeds. A gastric tube directly into his stomach has replaced it. Last Wednesday, Daniel had surgery to replace the bone flap in his skull that had been removed during the original surgery. All went well and he's doing fine. However, it was a shock to see him completely shaven again. His hair had started growing in nicely, giving him a more normalized look. As Joel keeps reminding me, Daniel's hair or lack thereof is the least of his problems.

We've settled into a routine. Joel goes to the hospital to visit Daniel some time in the morning, often at 11:00 a.m. when visiting hours officially start, but at times it's earlier if that's more convenient. Because Daniel's in a private room, no one complains. My part-time leave of absence started on October 18. I work every morning and spend every afternoon with Daniel. Usually, I bring along work to do for the times when he's sleeping or when the nurses are busy with him. One of us tries to visit in the evening, but we also rely on friends and family to spell us. Alyssa comes home as often as she can on weekends and Jonathan visits several times a week.

Daniel is awake most of the day, but his alertness fluctuates. He's usually most responsive in the morning and in the evening. He's certainly recognizing people and responding to many elements within his environment; however, his responses are still inconsistent when directions are given. Joel seems able to get the most from him. Perhaps it's the no-nonsense voice of a father that a child knows he must listen to. Jonathan says Daniel knows I'm a pushover so he just ignores me. He usually listens to Jonathan.

Our time with Daniel is spent trying to stimulate him in as many ways as we can. We have brought in the most recent family album and have plastered his wall with photos of his friends. The camp director has loaned us the 1993 album that Jonathan and Daniel's camp friends use to draw on memories from the summer. We have recently started showing him pictures from *Sports Illustrated* and *Ski Canada* magazines. The latter is particularly effective as he'll usually respond by moving his left leg as if he were skiing. Car magazines will be next, as he loves cars!

Television continues to hold his attention as it did in his pre-injury life. I think my mother was quite lucky to get a response of recognition when she arrived in his room the other day while the TV was on. Because he's still not talking, he doesn't protest when we turn it off.

The occupational therapist has started taking him downstairs to her department. Today, for the first time, Daniel differentiated objects by colour, and chose appropriately when asked. We're encouraged to see some movement in his right arm and hand, and supplement the exercises done by the physiotherapist with friends helping out on a daily basis. His right leg is still not moving on its own, but he does have sensation in his right foot. Daniel is showing greater dexterity with his left hand. He is now able to use a pincer grasp of his left thumb and forefinger to hold a feather or the stem of a leaf. The occupational therapist has told us to be encouraged when we observe Daniel executing purposeful movements, such as scratching his ear or his armpit or picking his nose. (I ask you, can a mother really be happy that her child is picking his nose and flicking it?)

We're still being told to focus on Daniel's current functioning on a day-to-day level, and not to anticipate the future or any prognosis. Boy, is this a tough order. How can we keep from wondering what he'll be like one or two years from now? The occupational therapist has told us that changes can continue to occur past the two-year mark and that his youth and the tremendous support he is receiving should aid in his recovery. However, behind all the hope that we're trying to muster is the realization that Daniel has sustained severe head trauma to the most important area of his brain.

Last week, one of the nurses asked if I would like to meet

"Steve," a young man who was a former patient at Sunnybrook Hospital. Steve had also been in a car accident and had been in the same room as Daniel is in now. Steve's father explained that the doctors had given Steve a dreadful prognosis including being unable to walk. He assured me that with his son's spirit, they were expecting a full recovery. Steve walked with a cane, talked, answered questions, etc. He had been at Sunnybrook for six weeks and was still at Riverdale, a rehab centre. His accident was thirteen weeks ago. While I was happy to see what can transpire, I was also discouraged by the slowness of Daniel's recovery. I know each person's progress is unique so we search for every possible response and change to indicate that progress is occurring.

Please continue to send us your cards and letters of support. We really appreciate hearing from you.

With love,
Lainie

CHAPTER SEVENTEEN

When the mail comes one Friday in mid-November, there it is — the letter I've been anticipating. My psychology exam results. Holding the envelope with trepidation, I hesitate before opening it. It's been four weeks now since the test, and the exam itself passed in a flash after all those months of intensive preparation. There were about one hundred candidates writing the exam that day, seated two by two at long tables in a hotel conference room, and the only familiar face was that of my colleague, Melissa. Afraid of distracting each other, we decided not to sit together. Platters of fruit and Danish adorned two tables at the sides of the room, and alongside them were large coffee urns and tidy rows of cups.

Who would take the time to eat in the middle of a four-hour-long exam? I thought.

Finishing early, I looked around at the other heads still bent in action, wondering if I had answered impulsively. I tried to check over my responses, especially those questions that stymied me with the possibility of two equally correct options. Yet with thirty minutes still to go, I handed in my booklet and left, heading directly to the hospital to visit my son.

Now as I carefully unfold the letter, the word "Congratulations" leaps out at me.

Racing for the phone, I call Joel and my mother, my words tumbling out in excitement. Then I leave a breathless message on Alyssa's answering machine and a quick note for Jonathan. I want to share my good news with Daniel too. That I'll have to do in person.

When I step into his hospital room, my nose crinkles in disgust. It takes only a moment to recognize that my son is preoccupied. Brown streaks are smeared over his shirt and the sheets like some abstract painting. My joy deflates instantly. I try to restrain his left arm while I wait for a nurse to change his diaper and clean him up.

Clump. Clump. Clump. My footsteps echo my dejection as I walk towards the elevator. The doors open. Swoosh. They glide to a close with a ding. Every sound reverberates in my head as if the volume has been amplified with extra speakers. My car engine roars as I wait in line to leave the garage. There's no special exit for monthly pass holders, and today there's only one cashier on duty. Finally I escape, and head northbound on Bayview Avenue.

I'm not sorry to have a shortened visit with Daniel, as I must attend teacher interviews for Jonathan. Murals brighten the hallways of his junior high school, but my tread is as nervous as if I were about to write another exam. Outside room 209, I squirm in a plastic chair and rub the knuckles of my left hand while waiting my turn. The geography teacher calls my name and I enter the map-covered classroom. Slowly he drums his fingers along the edge of the desk, peering at the file in front of him.

"When a student fails a test in my class, he or she is given the opportunity to rewrite it. Jonathan failed the first test in September and did nothing about it."

I can't believe it. Jonathan never mentioned anything. I expected that he wouldn't be putting forth great effort because of the crisis we've been in, but I didn't anticipate this.

"Is there no system in place to inform the parents?" I ask.

"Mrs. Cohen, your son is in grade nine. He must show responsibility for his own actions. I certainly don't have time to phone each parent when a student fails a test."

"But we're having a particularly difficult time in our family right now. I spoke to the guidance counsellor when school started. Didn't she say anything to you?"

"No, she didn't. All I know is that Jonathan is a new student in our school and his work is definitely below our expected standard. You'd better discuss it with him."

I leave room 209 and go down the hall to the math classroom. The news here is little better.

"Jonathan seems to have an attitude problem. He isn't focussed in class and his homework isn't complete."

There's no warmth, no understanding. No mention of our crisis, and I can't bring myself to raise the issue again. I leave the room, feeling confused and upset. Didn't the guidance counsellor relay the information I gave her? She said she'd take care of it, even offered to give Jonathan counselling support. I resolve to speak to her again on Monday.

I think of my son. How quiet he's been lately, polite yet removed. He spends so much time alone in his room, supposedly studying. What's he really doing? I used my exam studies as a way to avoid thinking of Daniel. Jonathan escapes from our harsh reality by playing basketball and watching television. Yet he had done so well last year in all his subjects, even working on an enriched math curriculum. I wonder how we can help him refocus on his schoolwork.

Home: another discovery. Above the French doors of our dining room waves a computer-generated banner with "CONGRATULATIONS" in big lettering. In the bottom right-hand corner of the sign, Jonathan has drawn a small book titled: *The Book of Brains by Little Mom*. I'm so pleased when he comes bounding out to greet me. He's carrying a chocolate cake with the message, "Congrats, Lainie," scrolled across the top in pink icing. My mom follows him from the kitchen and gives me a hug.

I won't talk to him now about school, I decide. My mother doesn't need to hear this. She has enough on her plate without worrying about this too. Besides, I'd like to savour this moment. We'll have time over the weekend for that discussion.

Late that afternoon Joel, Jonathan, and I drive up north to our cottage. It's our first visit back there since Daniel's injury and a typical November day. The sun, too weak to assert itself, disappears early in the leaden sky. The trees have shed most of their leaves and their barren branches wave at us with long skeletal fingers. I turn on the radio and flip through the stations trying to find something appealing.

"Hey stop, I like that," Jonathan pipes up.

Joel and I can't cope with the pounding bass and screeching lyrics. Quickly, I turn it off, then broach the topic of school, reporting what I heard in the interviews that afternoon along with my plan to contact the guidance counsellor.

"Why didn't you tell us you were having trouble?" Joel asks. "You could have retaken that geography test." His tone, without meaning to, sounds more accusing than solicitous.

I glance back at my youngest child, curled into the seat as if he'd like to disappear. I'm concerned about him. What a change from the bounciness he displayed earlier today.

Jonathan says nothing. Nothing at all.

Perhaps he's thinking, "What's the point in saying anything? There's nothing they can do. Even the guidance counsellor hasn't done anything. Besides, nobody can do anything to change Daniel and that's the real problem."

We continue our drive in silence.

In town, we stop to rent a pickup truck to transport the leaves on our property to the local dump; a new bylaw prohibits burning them. Jonathan settles into the cab beside Joel and I follow alone in our car. It reminds me of the time when we moved from our cottage on Pine Needle Point to our current place. That truck was a boxy six-ton rig with heavy tires. Jonathan had to hoist himself up to get into the front seat. He was only seven years old then, tall and thin with big gold-rimmed glasses. I expect he chattered to Joel non-stop, mostly about plans for a new tree house. He couldn't understand why the one we had built was not being moved along with our furniture and other belongings. I knew I'd miss it too. Miss seeing him climb up to the top with a knapsack of books, turning the pages of worlds filled with wonders.

It was strange watching my husband behind the wheel of that rig. He's such a slim man, not my image of the drivers I often see at truck stops or donut shops — men whose thick forearms flex with muscles and tattoos, whose heavy bellies dangle over their belts; men who seem to leave their worries behind when they smile and joke with the waitresses they meet. Yet Joel seemed comfortable, at home with the heavy clutch and multiple gears, perhaps enjoying the feeling of control, of mastery over a machine.

The cottage is cool and damp when we arrive. My husband starts a fire in the wood-burning stove in the family room and unpacks the car while I cook our meal. Like most of our recent dinners, this one passes quietly, and we soon settle ourselves in front of the fire. My brother offered to visit Daniel tonight and my thoughts are focused on the hospital despite the open book on my lap. Jonathan challenges his dad to a match of ping-pong and I'm delighted when Joel folds up his newspaper and accepts. It's been a long time since he's played with our youngest son.

Jonathan squeals with triumph when he wins a point. "Watch out, Dad. I'm going to whip your tail."

"It's not over 'til it's over, kid."

When they return, Joel shakes his head. "It's strange, almost like playing with myself. His style is so similar to mine. Won't be long now before he beats me."

I look at Jonathan, who is a clone of his father, and try not to think about Daniel. He wouldn't be here anyway, I remind myself. He'd be in the city, busy with his friends and his job.

The next day, the sky is again overcast, a thick foggy day of endless grey. We work outdoors, forming piles of rusted, crinkling leaves. So many leaves: maple, oak, alder, poplar, and birch, the crisp reds and oranges already fading to muted brown. I remember happier times of leaf raking. With kid-sized tools, our children used to help us gather the leaves into large cone-shaped piles that crunched and crackled when they'd leap into them. The yellows seemed so much brighter then, the reds more vibrant. Perhaps it was just the children's laughter that made them seem that way.

Today, damp clumps of leaves cling together, making the rake heavy in my arms, and I can feel the chill of winter coming. I'm grateful to pass on my tool when my nephews arrive with my brother-in-law to help. Back inside, I prepare some lunch, and while the pot of soup simmers and the casserole bakes, I have time to start writing up a report on a student I assessed this week.

It's already dark when David and the boys leave. Joel drives the truck back into town, and as arranged, slides the key under the locked door of the rental shop. On the way home, as we pass familiar sights, I wonder if we'll always relive that horrible night of Daniel's injury. I'm driving. Joel's head lolls against the back of the seat, his eyes drifting closed. His face looks drawn, more from accumulated worry than today's physical labour. How different from the happy times we shared in July, driving past the lush vineyards of the Loire Valley with its elegant châteaux. We had talked then about taking other travelling holidays, spending more time together, but for the past eleven weeks, all our time together has been spent in the hospital with Daniel.

After dropping Jonathan and the dog off at home, we head back to the hospital to find Daniel asleep in the dark with the TV on. Why are we here? Hoping that there's been some miraculous change since yesterday afternoon? I'm so weary. When Joel switches on the bedside light, Daniel's eyes open, but he doesn't turn his head towards us.

Suddenly, I feel angry seeing him lying there, unresponsive in this hospital bed. He brought this upon himself by not wearing a seatbelt. I know he didn't consciously choose this. This could never happen to him — seventeen years old and invincible. But it did, and we're all feeling the consequences.

Just then, Alyssa and her boyfriend drop in. My daughter looks so animated and energetic, the way a young person is supposed to be.

"Hey, what are you doing here? Aren't you both exhausted? Why don't you go home?"

Relieved, we nod, and as we step out of the room, we see Daniel's friend, Jaimie, approaching arm-in-arm with his girlfriend. A Saturday night date with a brief intermission for a hospital visit. What has happened to our Saturday nights? Friends continue to invite us to join them for dinners and shows, but we have little interest or energy. One day we accepted an invitation to brunch. In front of me a china plate with a silver rim, a water goblet, a mug, baskets filled with crusty bagels and rolls, plates of devilled eggs and smoked salmon, bowls of colourful salads. I observed the details like a stranger participating in some foreign cultural experience. The conversation swirled around me like an unfamiliar language, words that sounded alive, but held no meaning for me. I sat glued in place with a plastered smile, taking small bites, and wondering when we could leave.

Walking down the hallway to the elevator, I look at my husband's drooping shoulders and weary steps. I love my son, but resent what he's done to us. How will this all end?

On Sunday evening, to shake us out of our depressed state, I convince Joel to come to a movie with Jonathan and me. Munching popcorn and laughing at the silly antics on the screen, we manage to lose ourselves briefly in the celluloid fantasy of a Jamaican bobsled team. However, we can't resist the pull to stop by the hospital for another short visit on our way home, even though it's out of our way. Tonight Daniel has a bunch of friends visiting and seems very alert. The lively atmosphere of the group of guys feels almost party-like, and our spirits are buoyed once again.

A few days later, the speech and language pathologist meets me in the hallway. She explains her recent assessment of my son's swallowing and her continued concern about the protection of his airway.

"He's still not coordinating his breathing and the passage of air over his vocal cords to control sounds or cough voluntarily. This difficulty is a form of apraxia, and although his head control is improving, it still isn't at a consistently safe level for eating."

I feel like a kid on a seesaw partnered with someone heavier than myself who keeps me dangling up in the air. All my bouncing and jostling are helpless to dislodge it and bring me safely back to the ground.

CHAPTER EIGHTEEN

"Lainie, pick up the phone," Joel says, in late November. "It's Alyssa."

"Hi Mom. How's Daniel?" she asks, getting right to the point. Her daily question.

I picture her sitting cross-legged on her bed, bolstered with pillows, so far away in her university apartment. In the background, the muted voice of a soul-wrenching ballad. Joel and I answer, adding to each other's comments, layers of words about her brother, whom she hasn't seen for ten days now. Her attuned antennae pick up our anxiety about the slow rate of change.

"I'll be home again this weekend," she says. "He'll seem different to me."

Her voice now holds the honeyed warmth of summer and hammocks. I can't wait to see her. We cling to her hope, a life raft to keep us from drowning.

During her first year at university, she'd phone regularly with questions about laundry, recipes, and banking. Then the calls dwindled to once or twice a week, but they were chatty — anecdotes about new friends and discussion about her courses. Now with the focus on Daniel, it's hard to get her to talk about herself. We squeeze out information when she visits as we drive to the hospital or walk together from the parking lot. Her business courses start at 8:00 a.m. and she's swamped with work. I'm not sure how she manages to find time between classes to go to the pool three times a week. But she's having trouble with her shoulders. Before that it was her knees. Joint problems, the doctor suggested, uncertain of a distinct diagnosis. And the last time she visited, she mentioned scheduling an appointment with a counsellor on campus to help her deal with this crisis.

One evening months later, while I was preparing dinner, Alyssa came into the kitchen. She didn't offer to help. Instead she settled at the table nibbling a snack that I knew would ruin her appetite. Slouched in her seat, her shoulders hunched, she began to confide how she felt that night.

"When I hung up the phone, I turned up the volume of my stereo and lay down on my bed."

Chop, chop. Slices of carrots and curls of green pepper flew from my knife. I pictured my daughter hugging a pillow to her chest as the mournful strains of the singer's voice filled her room.

"Saturday night my roommate convinced me to leave the apartment. She pulled the book from my hands, 'C'mon, Lys. Enough already. Let's go out. There's a frat party at The Shot.'"

Seeing my raised eyebrows, Alyssa added, "It's a bar, Mom. I didn't really want to face that scene, but I didn't have any other plans so I went."

My vision changed to a scene of a crowded room with swirling smoke and pounding music. I knew not to interrupt.

"The rhythm thumped into my brain. Forget him, forget him, it seemed to say. Someone handed me a shot and then another. But it wasn't enough to erase Daniel's hospital bed. Nor the antiseptic smells filtering through the haze of cigarette smoke."

Chop, chop. The vegetables fractured into coloured streams of orange and green, lacing and interweaving in time to the beat.

"My hips swayed, but I didn't dance with anyone. In that crowded room, I felt so alone."

But that wasn't the whole story. It was almost four years later before I learned what Alyssa really felt. We were at a yoga retreat together attending a five-day grief workshop. We spent the first evening in a large carpeted room with the suffused glow of candles in the centre of our circle and soothing music in the background. Wide windows opened onto a vista of a grassy hill covered with bent apple trees. The leaders invited the participants to introduce ourselves by revealing not only what our loss was, but also a perceived victory and a challenge.

After my turn came Alyssa's. As she started to talk, she broke down in sobs. "I wanted to talk to you, really talk to you," she said to me, as if no one else in the room were listening. "But how could I tell you and Dad that I was as scared as you were? You were counting on me to be strong."

I cradled my daughter in my arms, hugging her, wishing that I could take back that heavy responsibility she felt burdened with. Later, Alyssa admitted that she assumed that role with the very first phone call to us at the cottage. She had censored also what the doctor had said to her when she signed the form for Daniel's surgery — your brother has a ten per cent chance of living. She couldn't bring herself to tell us how hopeless things looked, how close to death Daniel really was.

December 2, 1993
Dear Family and Friends,

A few days ago, I tried to write a newsletter to update everyone on Daniel's progress. I felt that I was listing events as if going through a checklist, but I wasn't capturing the flavour of what has been happening. My sister-in-law, Roz, excitedly claimed yesterday, "You're getting your son back!" In truth today I feel that we're starting to get back a new son, and I'm anxious to share the news.

When I went in to visit Daniel tonight, he was lying alone in the room covered by a sheet, but without any clothes on. (He usually wears a T-shirt and shorts.)

"What happened to your shirt?" I asked, and his response was an impish smile.

I sought out his nurse to solve this mystery and she explained that he had removed his shirt by himself. She had offered to put on a new shirt and he had refused, so she assumed that he was hot and would just remove the new one if she insisted. She also told me that she had asked him if he preferred to be called Daniel or Dan and he liked Dan.

I was agitated as I explained to my son that for eighteen years I have called him Daniel. Did he want me to change now? He nodded yes, but I didn't really believe it. I wrote both names on the Magnadoodle and he put a checkmark beside Dan. After I erased it, he took the pen in his left hand and printed: I WANT TO BE DAN!

Daniel had shown us that he could write names when asked, but until Tuesday he had not initiated writing any words on his own. This is really an incredible breakthrough! He has been using gestures to communicate and can often get his message across. Although he has started mouthing some words, he's still not talking at all. Now new vistas are opening up.

The biggest change is in his cognitive awareness. His level of comprehension has increased dramatically. He can consistently follow single-sentence directions and seems to understand much of what's said to him. Although he may be suffering from double vision, he has shown that he is able to read if the letters of words are written very large and thick.

Alison, the occupational therapist, has been concentrating on cognitive tasks that involve spatial perception, number recognition, short-term memory, and fine motor dexterity. Daniel has started showing more of his personality as he indicates that some tasks are too easy.

Let's get on with this, seems to be his recent message.

Alison has also measured Daniel for a rental wheelchair that will be customized to meet his needs. When he is more mobile, we will attempt to bring him home for a visit.

Jennifer, the physiotherapist, has been working daily with him to strengthen his head control and to help him sit erect in a "geri chair." Today, for the first time, he was moved out of bed by balancing his weight on his left leg instead of being hoisted up on a canvas with a Hoyer lift. He was so pleased with his success in standing, however brief the experience, and he has let us know that he wants to walk by making his fingers do the walking. However, his right side is still immobile.

Over the past several weeks, we've started playing familiar games with Daniel. When a game is first introduced, he requires modelling and support to play. Now he is able to play tick-tack-toe with strategy (he insists on going first and often wins). When playing "War" he recognizes which card is higher and either offers his card to his opponent or takes both in. He has even started playing euchre with his friends, but he needs a lot of help still. In the past few days, we've been able to introduce new activities at a much faster rate and he seems to be enjoying them: snakes and ladders, checkers, and Fabulous Fred (an electronic memory game). I've also started to read short stories to him. Whether it's the tone of my voice and the rhythm or the actual content that he's relating to, it's hard to tell, but he likes the experience.

Daniel's friends continue to visit, and the incentive they offer him just can't be duplicated. Last Thursday night, fifteen guys showed up in his room to celebrate his birthday. When they sang "Happy Birthday," he had a big grin on his face. However, when I asked him if his friends had good voices, he gave them a thumbs-down evaluation. He also tried to pull himself up in bed into a sitting position. Joel and one friend helped to support him while he held himself upright and looked around at the roomful of friends.

"Do you want a beer?" one friend asked.

My son's hand was immediately held palm up in anticipation of the fantasy bottle, and he sat with his head held high for longer than Jennifer had ever gotten him to do. What powerful motivators his friends are!

He's still not able to receive any food or drink orally, but he wants to. When we take him to the cafeteria to provide a change of scene, he will gesture that he wants to eat and drink too. One nurse explained to Daniel that his liquid feed is like a milkshake. Two days ago, he disconnected his feeding tube and was found trying to suck up the liquid from the tube that enters his stomach. This may suggest some purposeful action on his part, but a definite sense of confusion as well.

Following head injury, there are eight levels of cognitive functioning, and Daniel is now at Level IV. Confusion and agitation are features of his current level of cognitive awareness. He has demonstrated some inappropriate behaviour such as hitting, punching, and swearing with hand gestures, but we had been warned to expect these and to consider them a mark of progress. When he reaches Level V, he'll be eligible to transfer to a rehabilitation centre. He has been accepted into Hugh MacMillan Rehabilitation Centre and is on a waiting list. Hugh Mac has a special unit that caters to head-injured adolescents, and in addition to its fabulous reputation, it has the added advantage of being the closest rehab centre to our home. If Daniel is ready for rehab before a place becomes available there, he'll enter one of the other centres in Toronto on an interim basis (probably Riverdale, another well-reputed place).

We temper our excitement over Daniel's progress with the

knowledge that we don't know how far he'll go. It is possible to plateau at any one of the levels and even Level VIII does not reflect pre-injury functioning ability. But we're definitely hopeful that we'll see further progress. We'll keep you posted.

With love,
Lainie

The physiotherapist, occupational therapist, and nurses all offer advice for taking Daniel home. It's not a permanent leave taking, just a four-hour visit in early December, but an eager crowd gathers in the hall to watch us set off, and it feels momentous, like a ticker-tape parade. Somehow it seemed far easier to bring my son home as a squalling newborn from the hospital than it is this time. Or does memory serve me accurately? Mothers were not permitted to walk out of the maternity ward carrying their infants, and I remember Joel wheeling me to the door with our son bundled in my arms, then waiting for him to pull the car up to the entranceway and settle us in — me in the front and Daniel in his car seat in the back.

This time is different. Now it's Daniel's turn to be wheeled to the door, but he can't just step into a car. To eliminate the hassle of transferring him from his wheelchair into our car and back again, we've arranged for a taxi that's wheelchair accessible. Joel pushes the wheelchair to entrance B on the main floor, past the closed office doors that line the long hallway. The wheels roll awkwardly, constantly straining towards the right. We're like a rag-tag group of army veterans hobbling away from an action site. Our jackets spread across Daniel's lap, slipping and sliding towards the floor, and I follow closely behind, carrying a urinal, his communication binder, and a bag of dirty laundry.

It's a cold December day and I'm surprised to see several patients standing outside without their coats, bare legs exposed beneath hospital gowns, intravenous bags attached to metal poles, while they puff on their cigarettes as if gasping for their last breath. Not just smoke, but frosty air emerges from their lips in ragged white streaks that match the clouds in the sky.

In the doorway, I struggle to manoeuvre my son's right arm through his jacket sleeve; it's flexed too tightly against his chest and won't uncoil. Joel slides in Daniel's left arm and drapes the jacket over his right shoulder, and I bundle his head up with a hat and scarf, his torso and legs with a flannel blanket. Finally, I zip up my own jacket. Now we're ready.

Daniel is barely exposed to the fresh cold air as the taxi driver steps nimbly backwards, pulling him up the ramp into the mini-van. The wheelchair wheels are strapped in place and checked to ensure that they won't move. Then we're off. It's only a short drive, about ten minutes, and I'm grateful that the driver doesn't engage me in conversation. I watch my son gaze out the window. It's his first time in a car in almost four months. Does he recognize the familiar sights? The hockey arena where he spent so much time? The plaza where he and his friends would hang out in springtime at the ice cream store? Does he know he's going home?

There's a light dusting of snow on the wooden ramp that Joel and Jonathan built to fit over our three front stairs, and the going is slippery. The driver helps.

"You want me back in four hours? No problem, you can pay me then. Have a good time there, young fellow."

Bump.

"Just one more step. Easy now," I whisper, as if my words will smooth the wheels safely over the ledge.

The wheelchair is now over the threshold in our front hall. Alyssa and Jonathan crowd around while Echo barks at this strange metal contraption and shies away.

"It's okay, Echo," I say, gesturing the dog to come closer. Daniel dangles his left arm down to pat her and when he feels the top of her head, he smiles — a crooked smile, with just the left half of his mouth working its way into a grin.

Alyssa removes her brother's outerwear: his hat, scarf, jacket, and mittens, the reverse process faster than the original one.

"You're home, now, Daniel. It's great to have you here."

Away from the bright fluorescent lights in the hospital, there doesn't seem to be as much to him. The familiar muscular hulk that used to stride through these halls has shrunk by twenty-five pounds, and his pale face seems nothing but deep brown eyes, as dark as the inside of a cavernous well. He gazes at his sister briefly, and then his head tips to the right against his chair like a marionette with limp strings whose handler has disappeared from view.

Joel pushes the wheelchair through the wide hallway, past the "WELCOME HOME, DANIEL" banner that his brother has taped up, and through the narrow doorframe of the wood-panelled family room. Jonathan helps move aside the glass-topped coffee table so the coast is clear. Locking the wheels of the wheelchair in place, my husband unfastens the seatbelt, helps Daniel into a standing position and pivots him around. Alyssa moves the wheelchair out of the way while Joel gently lowers him onto the couch that I've covered with a flannel blanket.

My son's eyes are already closing. So much effort to get him here, just to have him fall asleep so soon. Still, it feels good to have all my children home again, if only for a few hours.

CHAPTER TWENTY

"Mrs. Cohen, telephone call, line one," the school's P.A. system announces with a scratchy sound.

"May I take this call here?" I ask the special education teacher. It's afternoon recess in mid-December and the two of us have been reviewing the test results of a grade four student whose papers are spread out on the table before us.

"Sure, go ahead."

Joan gathers the papers as I walk over to her desk, wondering about the caller. It's unusual for me to receive phone calls when I'm working in schools. Most calls come to my office and the secretaries there take messages for me.

"Hello. Elaine Cohen, here."

"Lainie," my husband's voice sounds distraught.

My breath catches. "Is Daniel all right?"

"He's fine. Just listen. It's about Jonathan."

I lean against the desktop, my eyes sweeping past the winter scene on the calendar to rest on the glass container of jellybeans. Near the top float two black ones, licorice-flavoured, my favourite.

"I just got a call from the principal at his school. Jonathan is in her office. There's been an incident."

"What happened? Is he okay?"

"Something to do with drugs. I'm going over to the school now."

"I'll come, too."

"No, don't. I'm much closer."

My husband's voice resumes its take-charge, no-nonsense tone. "I don't know what's going on, but I'll see if I can sort things out. You'll probably have a message at your office from the principal. Don't worry. You can ignore it. I'll call you later."

Don't worry. As if I could follow such advice. I replace the receiver and turn around. Joan's been busy with some files and now looks up at me, inviting conversation, an explanation for the missing part of the telephone exchange that she couldn't help hearing. For a moment I imagine myself leaning against her ample shoulders and sharing the news, but pride and my need to maintain a professional demeanour are too strongly ingrained.

"Family crisis," I tell her. "I'll have to leave early."

"Don't worry." Those dreaded words again. "We've finished what I needed. When I set up the parent interview, I'll let you know."

Her eyes continue to invite confession as I pack up my briefcase. I try to make my cracking voice sound jaunty.

"See you next week."

In the staff room, I retrieve my coat and boots. The recess bell must have rung although I didn't hear it. All the teachers have returned to class. There's no one to see my stricken face and ask caringly, "What's wrong?"

As I drive home, I think about this news. I can't understand it. Jonathan and drugs? He's only fourteen. With all our discussions about the dangers of drugs, we didn't think he'd get involved. And why now? Is this a bid for attention? His way of crying out? I haven't seen him cry even once since his brother's injury over three months ago.

We know this whole thing is hard on him. We know he must be hurting and we keep trying to talk to him, but when we ask him about school or friends, he replies in monosyllables, cutting us off. At dinner he eats quickly and quietly, anxious to leave the table and clear his place while we're still eating. He doesn't want to listen when we rehash the day's events at the hospital, tell of encounters with doctors, nurses, and therapists, share snippets of hope and feelings of despair. And he's still reluctant to visit Daniel, preferring to go to the hospital with Alyssa when she's in town, rather than with us.

A few days ago, when I took him with me, he held up photos from camp and started talking to Daniel.

"Here's one of you and Phil. Two cool dudes, eh? Remember the opening night for the Olympics? Boy, were those torches hot. Look at the sweat dripping from Phil when he took it, running all the way down the path to that huge bonfire. When they called out the teams

I got yellow. I'm always stuck on the yellow team and I never have anything to wear. I had to borrow someone's yellow bandanna. Remember? Because you lose points if you're not wearing your colour. You were on the blue team. It won, of course. I wish I'd been on the blue team, too."

Then he fell silent, watching his silent older brother in a hospital bed. Not the brother he knew; the one he's always tried to emulate and please. No, not his brother at all.

Pulling into the driveway, I approach the house and fumble with the key in the lock. The dog barks briefly, then quiets down when she hears my voice. I place my briefcase on the floor and bend down to pat her. She whines, as if saying, "C'mon, take me out. I've been waiting here by myself all day."

I sigh and let her out. It's not just Jonathan who's missing our attention. Daniel used to walk the dog every day. I'm not sure if Jonathan still does, although I remind him when I think about it.

I look out the window at Echo. She still looks like Lassie, the classic lines and sable colouring of a collie miniaturized to Sheltie size. I remember when she was a year-and-a-half old and Daniel was ten. It was February and a lot of snow had fallen that winter. Mounds of crusty snow banks were piled up against the curbs, browning at the edges in squishy slush that the cars sprayed as they passed. There were few sidewalks in our suburban community, so we had to walk Echo on the road. At least that's the way Alyssa and I did it. One day, I watched through the window in amazement as Daniel and Echo raced up and down every snowbank. Thirty minutes later they returned and collapsed in a wet heap of matted fur and soggy snow pants.

"Echo and I were defending Earth against space invaders. We won!"

Daniel's cheeks were rosy and cold. The bangs peeking out from his woollen toque were plastered against his forehead. As I bent over to dry his hair, he brushed aside the towel impatiently. Later, Echo flopped beneath his chair in the kitchen. Swinging his feet, he would rub against her back as he blew on his hot chocolate and spooned melted marshmallows into his mouth.

I call Echo back into the house. Has she got fatter? Her coat is much shaggier than usual. I can't recall the last time I brushed her.

When Jonathan enters the house, his glasses fog up and he wipes them off with his fingers. His face is pale and his shoulders are hunched over as if weighted down with a heavy knapsack, although his sits lightly on his back. Removing his school bag, he goes to the closet to hang up his jacket.

Joel comes in and slams the front door shut.

"What an awful experience. Seeing our son sitting with two cohorts outside the principal's office like three suspects in a line-up."

"Tell me what happened," I ask Joel.

My husband holds up his coat. I take it from him as he places his rubbers neatly on the mat. Jonathan slinks by and goes upstairs to his room. I don't greet him.

"I want to change first. Come upstairs and I'll talk to you."

I follow Joel to our bedroom. The oak furniture lends a solid feel to the room, and above the carved headboard in gold velvet mats are the professionally taken photographs of our three children as infants. Sitting at the edge of the bed, I watch my husband undress. He smoothes his suit pants along the crease, secures them evenly on the hanger and hangs up his jacket, then he places his tie on the rack, aligning it with the other blue ones that coordinate with his navy suits. Bunching up his white shirt, he shoves it inside the cabinet on his side of the bed and stomps back to the cupboard, where he quickly slips on a pair of corduroy pants and a flannel shirt. As he buttons his shirt, he finally turns to me. The words spew from his mouth.

"Jonathan and his friends were caught with a joint."

"In school?" I ask.

"No, in the park behind the fence. A teacher saw them, rounding up the stragglers after the lunch bell rang."

"I can't believe he'd try it."

"Turns out it wasn't the first time."

"What are you talking about?"

"Remember how pleased we were that Jonathan knew some students at this new school?" Joel asks.

"Yes." We'd been worried about him being a newcomer. With some familiar faces from camp and hockey, he seemed to have fit right in.

"Well, two weeks after classes started, Jonathan was at a party where some of these kids were smoking pot," Joel says, pacing the room.

"We taught him to just say no. He could have called us to get him." Even as I say these words, I picture us lying on the couch like zombies or crumpled in our bed. Two weeks after school started, Daniel was still in a deep coma.

Joel's angry voice breaks into my thoughts. "Hey, no one forced him. Jonathan says he was curious. But he had a horrible coughing spell and decided once was enough."

"Thank goodness. He could have had an asthma attack. I'm glad he didn't push his luck."

"Well, it seems he did. A few weeks later he tried it again."

"Why? Why would he do that?" I ask, shrugging my shoulders in disbelief.

"Says he wanted to be like the other guys."

I remember the conversation that Jonathan and I had about his friends. How he just wanted to shoot hoops with them and not think or talk about Daniel or school or anything else.

I tap the bedspread beside me, inviting my husband to settle down. "Where did the boys get the joint?"

"Are you sure you want to know?" Abruptly Joel gets up and walks around the bed. Picking up a pen from his night table, he flicks it open and shut.

"Of course, I do." I look at him expectantly, with my hands clenched against my belly.

He stops in front of the window, looks at the pen in his hand, and then at me. "From one of Daniel's friends."

"What? That's crazy." Now I'm standing too and wobbling a little, caught off balance by this remark.

"You know how Daniel's friends would always hang around the house, playing basketball and street hockey. Well, Jonathan got to know them well. Gave him status, being Daniel's younger brother. They called him 'Little Cohen' and sometimes they'd let him play with them."

"Right. So how could they do this?" I join my husband at the window. The curtains are drawn, holding back the darkness, and the brass chandelier over the bed twinkles with light.

"Jonathan says he asked a few guys and they brushed him off. Told him to forget it. He's too young. Stay away from drugs."

"That's what I'd expect. So what happened?"

"You know how persistent Jonathan can be. He kept bugging them."

"Now what?" I ask, wrapping my arms around Joel.

He returns my hug distractedly, then disengages. "Now we go and eat dinner and talk about something else."

In the morning, Jonathan leaves for school as usual, meeting up with a friend a few doors away. I still haven't spoken to him about this incident. I can't bear to be faced with his silence. I feel betrayed and afraid too. Afraid that my simmering anger will erupt and scorch us both. Better to remain silent.

Joel and I head off too. He'll visit Daniel before going to his office and I'll go there after work. The normal routines of daily life resumed, as if our current life can be considered normal.

At lunchtime I phone Joel. "Any news?"

"Yes, another call from the principal."

"What now?" I ask, bracing myself.

"She talked of suspending Jonathan."

"Can't we do anything? Speak to our school trustee or the superintendent and explain the circumstances? Jonathan's been under tremendous emotional stress."

It reminds me of the time when he was in grade three and hadn't done well in French class. Anticipating that the teacher would call and complain, he got on his bike and ran away, leaving behind a cryptic note. It took us hours before we found him, playing calmly at a friend's house in our former neighbourhood, miles from where we had recently moved. I was overwrought. Tears brimmed as I hugged him, my fears and relief so intertwined. We listened then, hearing his unspoken plea.

"Maybe this is just his cry for help."

"I explained all that and the principal is sympathetic. She'd really like to help, but the school board has a policy of zero tolerance for drugs and violence."

"Can't she do anything at all?"

"She has a meeting scheduled with the superintendent on Monday. However, she's not optimistic. The guidelines are clear. She expects he'll be suspended for twenty days."

"What will happen? Will he lose his year?" I ask, shuddering at the thought.

"She assures me that she doesn't want him to be punished academically. The guidance counsellor will speak to all his teachers and arrange for school work to come home."

"We can't count on that. We'll have to hire a tutor to help him out."

"Right now that sounds like the least of our worries."

The next few days are like walking around a large statue that someone has installed right in the middle of our kitchen. We can't avoid it. Its bright bronze sheen glares as if daring us to touch it. I can barely look at Jonathan. When I do catch his eyes, they quickly dart away.

"Why did you do this?"

My youngest son remains silent.

"Did you think about us at all? There we were at the hospital every day with your brother still in a coma. So tired at night that we'd collapse into our bed. We trusted you."

I feel so resentful, the words rush out like cutting knives. I want them to shatter his exterior calm, his hard shell. This sullen fourteen-year-old seems impossible to reach. Perhaps I would sound more empathic if he expressed remorse, admitted poor judgement or wrongdoing. Yet he remains silent, challenging us to love him anyway. Unconditional love. Isn't that what parents are supposed to give? No matter what the child has done — condemn the behaviour, not the child.

Notice me — his unspoken message. You're so engrossed in my brother, it's almost as if I don't even exist.

Maybe that's what I'd like to believe he was thinking. Would I have reacted differently if he had said it was just a casual experiment? If he had told me, "It's nothing serious, really, Mom. There's no need to get upset."

Would that have changed our response? I doubt it. I remember what happened two summers ago when we brought Jonathan up to the cottage one weekend with three friends. The boys were so excited as they set up their stuff in the guest cabin. But the excitement didn't last long. When Joel opened the screen door to invite the boys for a boat ride, he caught the glittering sheen of something being stashed under a pillow.

"What's that?" he asked.

"Oh, nothing."

Joel strode over to the bed and picked up the pillow, exposing a cigarette lighter. "Let's see what other nothings you've brought."

Reluctantly the boys emptied their knapsacks. Joel confiscated a pack of cigarettes, two books of matches, a bottle of vodka, a knife, and a *Hustler* magazine.

Maybe he should have left it at that and returned the goods at the end of the weekend. Laughed it off, as boys will be boys. Maybe he shouldn't have told me. But he did, and we decided it was better to nip things in the bud. Teach them a lesson, we thought. Consequences for their actions. So we called each of the parents, explained what had happened, and arranged for the boys to go back to Toronto the next morning. We always felt we had done the right thing.

I later wished that I had responded differently when Jonathan first came in from the principal's office, that I had immediately wrapped my arms around him. What Jonathan felt was my silent anger — anger masking my fears and my powerlessness to keep my children safe from harm. Simmering rage that I couldn't express about Daniel's injury found a fault line seeking release. When I did finally reach out and pulled him towards me, his thin body stiffened in my arms.

"What's going to happen to us?" I ask my youngest son.

Joel, Jonathan, and I drive to the social worker's office. The evening air is crisp and I burrow my gloved hands into the pockets of my coat. It takes a while for the car to warm up. Glittering lights on trees and houses announce the upcoming holiday season. We pass by the office building before I make out the address.

"Turn here, into the plaza," I tell Joel.

He makes a quick right turn. The plaza is small, with only half a dozen stores. The grocery, pharmacy, and bank are all closed. Only the video store is open, with its catchy posters and flashing neon sign, but the frosted windows obscure any customers. I'm glad I'm not alone.

My husband parks the car and we head towards the office entrance at the end of the plaza. Jonathan drags his feet.

"Hurry, it's cold out here," I say.

"Let's take the stairs. It's only one flight up," Joel says. He's already halfway up as he makes the suggestion, eager to get this whole thing over with.

The initials on the door indicate the primary occupant of the office, a lawyer who works here by day. We knock and enter the empty waiting room.

"Is that a closet?" I ask, but don't bother to check. I fold my coat in my lap. Joel sits beside me on the couch and places his jacket alongside. Jonathan sits alone on a chair. I wonder what they're thinking. They look so alike sitting there with their arms crossed against their chests, their right fingers slowly squeezing their left forearms. Jonathan hasn't expressed his thoughts to us or to Alyssa either. Not that I'd expect her to betray his confidence if he did talk to her, but somehow she would find a way to reassure us if he had.

Leaning against the back of the couch, I clasp my hands over my stomach. It's my weak spot. Whenever I'm upset, my stomach is too. The wait seems interminable.

A woman emerges from the inner office to greet us. Her long skirt is flowing like her wavy auburn hair. A colourful shawl is draped around her shoulders, more for style than for warmth.

"Please, come in. Sorry to keep you waiting. Why don't you hang up your coats?" she says, gesturing to the closet. "You'll be more comfortable that way."

Reluctantly, Jonathan unzips his ski jacket and follows us into the inner office. The therapist settles herself opposite us as we sink back into the soft cushions of the black leather couch.

"I'm going to take notes as we talk," she tells us. "First I'll need some background information."

The hour goes by quickly; Joel and I do all the talking.

"Perhaps it would be better if next time I see your son by himself. Would that be all right with you, Jonathan?"

His nod is barely perceptible.

"How about this Thursday at the same time? I expect we'll see each other once a week after that."

Her smile is warm and inviting. His look is stony and blank.

CHAPTER TWENTY-ONE

I remember the summer Jonathan was five, his cowlick of fine blond hair fluttering like a flag in the breeze, the first summer we spent in our cottage by the lake. I thought he might find it lonely with his brother and sister away at sleepover camp for three weeks. But Jonathan delighted in my undivided attention and loved having the children from next door to play with. There were other playmates too — two little boys he met at the community beach where swim lessons were held three times a week. When their lessons ended, the boys would run through the woods together or play with action figures in the sand.

One late afternoon, we were surprised to see a woman arrive at the beach with two small white goats. Frolicking at the edge of the water, the goats kicked up sand with their heels and butted their heads into one another. Jonathan and his friends pranced nearby and mimicked their actions.

An unexpected growl splintered our laughter. A brown dog appeared from out of nowhere, it seemed, and raced down to the water. Its ears were flat against its head and its teeth flashed white as it tried to corner the goats, snapping at their heels. The frightened goats bumped into each other, skittered into the woman who stood helplessly by, then leapt frantically one after the other onto a picnic table.

"The dog's hurting them," wailed Jonathan. He ran to my side.

"No, he's just trying to herd them together. He thinks that's his job. They'll be okay."

We withdrew as the dog circled the table, pawing the air. Its snarls reminded me of the pack of mutts near our old cottage, the ones that roamed free and terrorized any passers-by with their snappish manner and infernal yowls. We never learned if they bit or not. Our family always avoided that road.

"I never want a dog," Jonathan said, climbing into the safety of our car.

But it was too late — we had already set the wheels in motion. For years Daniel had been yearning for a dog. Now we planned to surprise him with one when he returned home from camp.

A week later, when I pulled up in front of the breeder's house, Jonathan was with me.

"I'll wait in the car," he said, slumping deeper into the seat near the rear window. I took him by the hand and gave a little tug.

"C'mon."

Soon the two of us were standing in front of a thick wooden door with a door knocker in the shape of a woodpecker's head. Barks and yelps followed the tap, tap sounds.

"I don't want to come," Jonathan said, burying his face into my side.

I patted his head, smoothing down his cowlick. "Shhh, it will be okay, you'll see."

The lady who answered the door had a cheery voice that trilled, "Hi, I'm Jane. Come on in. The puppies are waiting for you."

Jane led us across a green-carpeted hallway to a closed door, then down a flight of stairs. The pungent smell of puppy urine assailed our nostrils. My son gripped my hand even harder. The wood floor was covered with sheets of newspaper and in the corner of the room was a large fenced-in area with five puppies, white and tan balls of fur that yapped and jumped up on the mesh of the cage.

"Why don't I introduce you to the mother first? Chelsea's in the next room."

Chelsea looked regal with long thick fur and a big white ruff, her brown eyes darker than rich dark chocolate. I bent down and scratched her ears. When Chelsea went to sniff Jonathan, he jumped back, tucking his hands in his pockets.

"Oh, what a gentle dog," I said. "She's lovely."

"Chelsea's mother and father have won all kinds of prizes and she just won her first blue ribbon. Most of her pups are show-quality dogs."

"We're not interested in showing a dog. All we want is a good pet."

Jane opened the door to the cage. Four of the puppies bounded out and scurried across the wooden floor, landing at our feet. They clamoured for attention. Choose me, choose me, they all seemed to say.

It was too much for my youngest child. He jumped onto a chair and waved his hands around like a whip, a nervous lion tamer escaping from the wild beasts out of control below him.

He watched as I picked up a pup and cuddled it in my arms. It nuzzled against my chest and licked my chin. When I carried it towards Jonathan, he held up one hand like a police officer stopping traffic.

"That's close enough."

Gently, I returned the pup to the floor and flipped it over onto its back. Its four legs bicycled in the air.

"Sorry, pal, you won't do. We really wanted a female dog."

"You won't have much choice then," Jane said. "I'm keeping this one to breed and that one has already been spoken for." She pointed to an active pup that was trying to climb the leg of the chair. "The only other female is the puppy still in the cage."

We looked towards the cage at the puppy that seemed so much quieter than her brothers and sisters.

"I don't think we'd want a nervous dog," I said, glancing over at my son who still stood on the chair.

"Oh, she's fine, really, she's just a little shy. Come here, sweetie," she called. The pup scampered out of the cage towards Jane. "I'll crate the others so you can have a chance to play with her."

The shy puppy played near my feet. After a few quiet moments,

Jonathan climbed down from the chair. The puppy looked as if she had a fluffy white scarf wrapped around her neck, white tube socks on all four paws and a smudge of white chalk in the centre of her nose. Her ears flipped up and over and her dark eyes shone like the bright button eyes of his favourite teddy bear. I smiled as he took one step closer and then another. Bending lower, he gingerly patted her back. So soft, so small, not scary at all.

It will be okay, I thought. It will definitely turn out all right.

CHAPTER TWENTY-TWO

At the start of the winter holidays our friends, Al and Marilyn, invite us to join them at their chalet for a few days of skiing. Joel encourages me to go with Jonathan.

"You're on holiday from work. Take advantage of it. I'll visit Daniel while you're gone."

"What about you? Maybe I should stay in the city and let you go with Jonathan."

"That wouldn't work. Daniel needs me to transfer him to the washroom right after breakfast. The nursing staff is so limited around Christmas, they'd never get to him in time. Besides, I'm not in the mood."

Am I in the mood? Do I even want to be alone with Jonathan

right now? Holiday time has always been family time. When Jonathan was six years old, we took the whole family skiing for the first time at Mont St. Anne, not far from Quebec City. Daniel raced on ahead to the lift line, while his younger brother clumped behind us, trying to get used to walking in his stiff ski boots. We started off slowly, and by the afternoon, Daniel was egging Alyssa on to ski ahead with him.

On the chairlift, Alyssa chattered about school and her friends, about what was happening in Brownies, gymnastics, and her ballet classes. Jonathan, wrapped tightly in his father's arms, his skis dangling between Joel's legs, piped in with his own comments and questions. Daniel sat quietly.

"What are you thinking about?" I asked.

"Nothing. Just watching them ski," he said, pointing to the expert skiers on the steep mogul run below us. At the top, he scooted off the lift to mimic what he had observed. Flexing and jumping, he and his skis almost disappeared, lost in the mounds like in a giant's cheeks bulging with a half-chewed child.

On our fourth day, the weather turned glacial. Blustery winds swooshed down the mountain, swirling snow into drifts. Jonathan seemed to move slower than ever. Each time we stopped, cold air renewed its attack, and soon my youngest child seemed to be playing frozen tag, waiting to be tapped before moving again.

"Swing your arms around. Big circles. You'll feel warmer," I said.

We could hear Daniel's impatient voice calling us from down the hill, but Jonathan stood rooted to the hillside, his lips shivering. I pulled his neck-warmer higher up and covered his nostrils. Frigid air blew in our faces and attacked every exposed spot — the top of our goggles, the back of our necks, our wrists where ski mitts and sleeve jackets separated.

"Let's go. We'll get some hot chocolate to warm you up."

At the top of the north side stood a small timbered hut with a large potbellied wood stove. We entered an atmosphere of steaming warmth, of tall aluminum pots that hummed with bubbling soup and spicy chilli. The cook took one look at Jonathan and immediately hoisted him onto an unlit burner, beside the pot of chilli. Jonathan sat there, sipping a hot chocolate, the colour slowly returning to his face, while I rubbed my hands together and tried to bring back the circulation to my blue-tipped fingers. There was still a long run back to the base of the mountain.

Jonathan travels north with Marilyn and her kids. Two days later I set off to join them. With little snowfall, the highway is clear and the traffic is light on this weekday morning. I put a cassette into the tape deck and soon find myself singing along, remembering the trip to New York that Alyssa and I took when she was fifteen. Aunt Selma and Uncle Howie picked us up at the airport and drove us straight to Manhattan, where we walked around like typical tourists crushed in the rush of the crowds, gawking at the tall buildings and window-shopping in the designer stores along Fifty-seventh Street, trying to imagine the type of outfits we'd need to accompany the nine-hundred-dollar Gucci purse we had just seen. Alyssa asked to do some real shopping in Bloomingdale's, and I was afraid she'd never want to leave, but at 6:00 p.m. as planned, we met our relatives for dinner. They had booked tickets to *A Chorus Line* and Alyssa was enthralled. Her first Broadway show!

Step, step, kick, kick. Alyssa and I have listened to this tape together countless times since then. I can feel the tap of the dancers' feet, hear the snap of their hats, still picture the bright sparkle of their vests, the glittering lights of the stage. Listening to the music puts me in the mood for a good time.

I place my skis over my left shoulder and walk through the parking lot over the wooden bridge to the ticket kiosk. There's Al, with his booming hello.

"Great timing. The kids just took a run and should be back at the chairlift by the time you're ready. Marilyn is at the clubhouse dealing with our picnic hamper. She'll meet us at the top."

"Whoa! Slow down. I'll just scoot to the washroom first. Looks like a great day. How are the conditions?"

"Pretty good for this time of year, although not all the runs are open. Yesterday Jonathan tried out Katie's snowboard."

"He did? How was it?"

"Well, he was back on his skis after only one run. He didn't think his right hip could take any more ground, but he had fun. He's a good skier and a great kid."

"Yes, he is," I say, turning aside. "Give me a minute. I'll be right with you."

It's just past 5:00 p.m. and the sky is darkening outside the chalet window. Inside, we're snug and warm, sprawled on couches and chairs around the fire. Sparks shoot off from the crackling logs. Hiss, zing. The sounds add to the chorus of voices that fade in and out. Jonathan and the two older girls are playing cards while the two younger kids play on the floor nearby. Al opens a bottle of wine and Marilyn brings out chips, cut-up vegetables and dip, smoked salmon, and crackers.

"Dig in, guys. You must be hungry," she says.

"Are you kidding?" I reply. "After the feast you served at lunch?"

Leaning back contentedly, I take a sip of wine and help make the food disappear. My muscles have a pleasant ache to them, enough to know they've been exercised, not enough to stop me from skiing again tomorrow.

"What a great day! And we'll have another one tomorrow," Al predicts. "The forecast is for sunshine. That should soften up those clumps of ice that were forming by late afternoon."

"Can't complain. We got in a full day." I stretch out my legs on the coffee table and wriggle my ankles.

"Hey, take that back," the youngest daughter whines. "It's not your turn. Daddy, he's cheating."

"No, I'm not. She never plays fair," her brother gripes.

"Stupid, now look what you've done. You flipped over the board."

I glance at Jonathan. Is he shuddering too? The whining voices are a painful reminder of how different our lives are now. Our house is so lonely and quiet with just Jonathan at home.

"I better get started on dinner," I say. "As hosts, you're entitled to sit back and be served. It will be ready in a jiffy."

I carry my wineglass into the kitchen and take out a large

frypan. As I start to chop the onions, I reach into my pocket for a Kleenex and dab my eyes. Soon the chicken is sizzling in the pan, taking on a crisp brown hue. The vegetables are all cut and ready to be added, a colourful assortment of greens, oranges, and reds, and on the back burner is a large soup kettle of bubbling water for the noodles. The hum of the voices and the children's laughter mingle with the sounds in the kitchen.

"Katie, could you take out a tablecloth please, and get Jonathan to help you set the table?" Marilyn asks.

The meal I serve everyone is delicious.

That night Jonathan and I lie in the basement in a twin-bedded room, talking quietly about snow conditions and skiing. It's nice to have a neutral topic to discuss, and I feel a bond with my youngest child. It reminds me of the time when he was five and Joel had taken Alyssa and Daniel away for a ski weekend. How empty the table looked with just two place settings for our Friday night dinner. Jonathan scurried to his room, returning with his arms brimming with stuffed animals that he carefully placed on pillows in each empty chair. Then he covered the heads of Teddy and Monkey with *kippot* in anticipation of the prayers while I set out more cutlery for our guests. I remember there was a warmth, a glow beyond the Sabbath candles that filled the room that evening.

"Do you want to ski tomorrow?" I ask.

"If you want to. Makes no difference to me," he answers, withdrawing into the silence that he now wears like a mask.

Tossing and turning, I try to find a comfortable position in the bed. The mattress sags in the middle and I can't seem to settle down. Despite the warmth of the comforter, I feel chilled. I can't imagine sleeping here another night. So I decide — tomorrow morning I'm going home. Jonathan can come with me or stay on if he prefers. One day away from Daniel is all I can handle.

January 4, 1994
Dear Family and Friends,

The rate of change that Daniel is undergoing seems incredible; so much has happened since my last newsletter. Yet even as I write these words I'm filled with trepidation, as we don't know if the changes will stop just as quickly and what the end result will be. He's now at Level V of the eight cognitive levels and will transfer to Hugh MacMillan Rehabilitation Centre on January 13.

Alison, the occupational therapist, was discussing the intense rehabilitation that will be taking place at Hugh Mac and asked him what he thought of the idea.

He shook his head and answered, "Too much work" — a typical teenage remark.

Daniel would probably classify passing the swallow test on December 22 as his most important accomplishment. He was given barium-coated food in different consistencies and X-rayed as he consumed them. The next day he started being fed soft food. We know he was disappointed, as he expected to get "real food" (a burger and fries would have been his choice). He wrote us a message: "This food not good." He ate every morsel anyway. He isn't allowed any bread or liquid yet, but we expect that will change shortly as his swallowing has improved significantly and another test will soon occur.

Eating is now the focus of his day and the topic of much of his communication. After finishing breakfast one morning, he asked for "another meal." When you consider that breakfast consisted of a poached egg, a bowl of rolled oats with brown sugar, applesauce, Jell-O, and gelled juice and coffee, you would have thought he had enough. But he wrote, "I'm near starvation!"

The introduction of food has brought a new set of expectations and adjustments. The nursing staff is stretched very thin, especially over the holiday period. Daniel's meals must be supervised to retrain him to feed himself and to ensure that he doesn't eat too quickly or too much and begin choking. Joel and I started to take turns to be with him at breakfast time, which means that our visiting hours extend from 8:00 a.m. to 9:00 p.m. instead of beginning at 11:00 a.m. However, a new stage, that is in fact a growth step for Daniel, has made me feel frustrated and powerless. After breakfast, he's begun to indicate that he needs to go to the washroom. Joel is able to take him, but my lack of height and upper body strength prevent me from trying to transfer my son, whose lack of balance could topple us both.

Daniel's right leg is becoming more mobile. He's now able to lift his leg off the bed and move his foot. When he is helped to a standing position, he'll balance on his right leg also. Although his right arm is slower to show improvement, there is some movement in his right thumb and fingers. Every change is a positive step towards greater independence.

Our son is just beginning to whisper words. His breath control is inconsistent and he really has to concentrate to whisper even softly, but we hope that he'll be talking soon. He seems to have a lot to say and has taken an interest in making phone calls. If you get a call and do not hear a hello, but hear beeps instead, don't hang up — it could be him. One beep stands for yes and two beeps for no. Yesterday he dialled a wrong number and the person on the other end thought there was a problem with his phone, what with all the beeping and no sound.

Daniel's personality is definitely re-emerging. The nurses think he's so sweet and polite. Visitors for other patients frequently stop to say hello and ask how he is. He'll smile and respond, "Fine," waiting until they walk away before quizzically gesturing, "Who are these people?"

On two occasions he has managed to con his friends into transferring him back to bed from his wheelchair.

"Shouldn't we call a nurse?" asked one.

"No, you do it!" Daniel emphatically mouthed as he pointed from the wheelchair to the bed.

He will need this assertiveness and determination to be successful in rehab.

We've brought Daniel home to visit several times for day visits. Once he's settled in rehab, he'll be coming home on weekends. This phase will bring new adjustments to our lives. It's both tremendously exciting and scary to anticipate.

The continued care and support of family and friends is incredible. Thank you.

Love,

Lainie

CHAPTER TWENTY-THREE

January 13, 1994. The big day has finally arrived — Daniel's transfer from the hospital to the Hugh MacMillan Centre. We've been waiting for this event since the day in late October when the director of Hugh Mac's brain injury unit came to the hospital to evaluate him.

I was as nervous as the mother of a four-year-old being interviewed for some posh private school, wanting my child to be on his best behaviour, praying he wouldn't pick his nose or worse. But it was not one of Daniel's better days.

The doctor impressed us by trying to engage directly with Daniel instead of talking over his head as if he weren't even there. However, Daniel was unresponsive and couldn't follow many of the doctor's instructions. As much as Joel and I tried to be quiet observers, we couldn't resist piping in now and then, "We've seen him do that. He really can do it."

When the doctor finished his examination, he turned and talked to us. My moist brown eyes gazed at him like a puppy begging for scraps.

"I've talked to the neurosurgeon who feels that Daniel is a good candidate for our facility." He paused briefly, cleared his throat, and then continued.

"I've decided to accept him, but we'll have to wait until he reaches Level V of the Rancho Los Amigos Scale before transferring. Right now, as you know, he's at Level III."

Our sighs of relief were distinctly audible, and Joel eagerly pumped the doctor's hand in thanks.

"Phone the centre and arrange for a visit. I'll let Bob, our social worker, know to expect your call."

When the doctor left, I turned to the window to re-read the chart we had posted on the nearby wall about the Rancho levels of cognitive functioning. Descriptions of awareness, orientation, and behaviour were clearly given for each of the eight levels. The only information missing was how quickly a patient would move from one level to the next. No one could tell us that. What was worse was the possibility that Daniel could plateau at a level and not move on at all.

Teary-eyed, I now stand in my son's hospital room. All the posters, photos, personal information sheets, and get-well cards are gone. Daniel's friend, Robert, helped Jonathan pack up the hockey shirt and trophies in boxes the night before. We carted them home along with the games, toys, magazines, and stimulation material we've been using. The room has resumed its sterile anonymity. Blank cream walls, a bed with rumpled linens that will soon be stripped clean, and a brown leatherette chair under the window. His home for so many months.

Daniel is fully dressed in sweatpants and a sweatshirt, ready to leave. Sitting in his wheelchair, he's making rapid walking gestures with his index and middle fingers and mouthing, "Let's go."

But we can't leave yet. Something's gone wrong.

His nurse this morning, a supply staff, hadn't noted that Daniel's liquid intake is restricted. She gave him water to drink instead of crushing his pills into applesauce or jam. Now a doctor must check that his chest is clear of fluid before it's safe to go.

While we're waiting, I offer to take a photo of him in front of his room. We position the wheelchair in the doorway so the room number is visible — C157. Will we ever forget it? I doubt that he'll remember. Just last week, the occupational therapist informed us that Daniel's orientation to time and place is still distorted. Sometimes he thinks he's in an office building and has no concept of the months that have passed since his injury.

When the Polaroid picture is ready, I show it to Joel. The camera has captured a spaced-out look in our son's eyes, as if he's staring into the distance but not really seeing.

"He doesn't look normal," Joel complains.

The photo has captured the reality that we're trying so hard to forget.

It's just a short drive to the rehab centre and the reception here is very smooth. Warmly greeted by two nurses, we're shown to a room directly across the hall from the nursing office. They invite Daniel to rest in bed and get him settled before tackling the comprehensive intake questionnaire with us. Joel and I sit in chairs skirting his bed beside a large picture window. Open curtains reveal a mound of snow outside the window ledge with the tips of some golden-green euonymus bushes barely visible. Just beyond are the bare branches of towering maples and oaks and some pine trees, whose dark green needles are heavy with snow. How soothing to have greenery to look at.

Across the aisle is the only other occupied bed in this large four-bedded room. Family pictures, posters, and get-well cards for its teenage occupant bring a sense of life to the surroundings. We'll soon decorate the bulletin board above our son's bed too.

The nurses' questions go on for a long time. Daniel dozes.

"Oh my, look at the time," one nurse says as she gently pats him awake. "We'd better get you some lunch."

She leaves the room, while the other nurse helps him transfer to his wheelchair. She straps him in. I look around to set up the tray table, but can't find any.

"We'll go to the solarium today," Maureen says. "Patients never eat in their rooms. That's one of our rules."

We wheel Daniel to the solarium, a wood-panelled room with two windowed walls. Dull clouds scud across the sky and a weak wintry light creeps in. In one half of the room are long tables and wooden chairs, cabinets, and a sink; the other half is filled with a well-worn couch with sagging cushions, a few easy chairs with fraying fabric, a large television set, and a bookcase with a stack of games.

"This is where the teenagers hang out. You'll get to know it well," Maureen says.

Right now the room is empty.

"The others are all in the dining room. When Daniel's been with us for a while, he'll get to eat there too."

Kris returns with a tray laden with food and places it at one end of a table. I wheel Daniel over and am about to settle down beside him when Maureen shoos me away.

"You two had better grab a bite to eat in the cafeteria before it closes."

So we leave our son under her watchful eye. When we return to his room after lunch, we find him back in bed with the side rails up.

Joel asks, "Do you need to pee?"

He replies, "I did already," and points to a spreading puddle on the floor.

We buzz for a nurse. Kris laughs when she finds out what he's done. "Good problem solving, young man. At least you didn't get the bed wet. I'll bring you a urinal and attach it to the bar here, where you can reach it for next time."

What a wonderful attitude! We like this new setting already.

Weekends — a new hurdle. As the first one approaches, we ask the medical director what to do with Daniel, expecting to be given a list of activities to pursue to reinforce the therapy he's been having.

"Do what you'd normally do. Be his parents, not his therapists."

Such simple advice seems like another insurmountable challenge. When we were all in the city together and not at the cottage or on vacation, what did we actually do with our teenage son before his injury? Not much. *Shabbat* dinners were a command performance that he was expected to attend, although he often rushed out to join his friends before dessert was even served, a source of never-ending annoyance to me. The rest of the time we saw little of him. When he was home, the door to his room was often closed with the music blaring. Either that, or he'd be huddled in front of the TV in the basement. If he were working on the weekends, he'd be out early; otherwise there'd be a hulking unshaven presence in the kitchen as he ate his first meal around noon. He didn't join us for cross-country skiing, for bowling, not even for movies anymore, although he was always happy to cadge a meal if we were going to a restaurant for dinner.

What are we supposed to do now? With Daniel at home on weekends needing constant supervision, we don't have time to pursue our own interests or even to catch up on the everyday errands that accumulate during the week. By late Sunday morning, claustrophobia hits; I'm being buried in stacks of dirty laundry.

"Let's go to the mall," I say.

It takes time to dress Daniel in outdoor clothing, transfer him into the car, dismantle his wheelchair, and repeat the process in reverse when we get there. Jonathan comes with us, enticed by the promise of food, but he wants to browse in the stores and check out the latest music releases. We pull him along. His brother is already tired and if we're to eat, we must do it quickly; there's no time for a relaxed meal in one of the restaurants.

Fast food outlets line the walls of the food court. The odours here coalesce in the uneasy alliance of rival countries: Chinese, Japanese, Greek, and Italian, as well as the standard hamburger joints. Joel stands in line at one kiosk, Jonathan at another. Plastic chairs are riveted in place and I try to find a clear space at the end of a table to position Daniel's wheelchair. I get him settled, then take out his gelled drink and a spoon from the carry-all bag. When my guys return laden with burgers, fries, salads, and slices of pizza, Daniel is already spooning his drink and drooling a little. His glazed expression glows at the sight of the golden fries.

Jonathan takes a seat and glances skittishly behind him. Perhaps in his mind the unasked question: what if there's someone here I know? Then, ducking his chin down, he lowers his eyes and starts to eat.

Meanwhile Daniel slowly masticates his mouthfuls like a cow chewing its cud. I nibble on my salad, push the excess dressing off to the side, then lean towards Daniel and wipe a dab of ketchup off his chin. I'm surprised to see my youngest already standing, his food completely gone, inhaled as if he were an industrial suction machine.

"I'll meet you back here. Going to check out the CDs on the upper level," Jonathan says.

By the time he's finished his meal, Daniel's head is lolling against the headrest of his wheelchair. We've no time to window shop or pick up the few things I need from the grocery store. We must take him home and put him to bed. As we push Daniel to the exit, Jonathan lingers behind, dragging his feet.

CHAPTER TWENTY-FOUR

It's January 29 today, a Saturday morning, exactly five months since Daniel's injury. Not a day for celebration, I think, as I turn off the alarm and reluctantly pull myself out of bed. Winter's darkness shrouds the bedroom although it's almost 7:00 a.m. I slip on some clothes and walk downstairs. Jonathan is already standing at the front door with his jacket on, his ski equipment on the floor beside him.

"Hurry, Mom. We're supposed to pick up the other guys at 7."

Mother-chauffeur: the two words are inextricably intertwined when you live in the suburbs. There's almost a relief when teenagers start driving themselves — but look where that's got us. I'm glad that Jonathan and his friends aren't old enough to drive yet. Thankful, too, that he'll be supervised in lessons today, not just skiing alone with his friends. He hasn't spent much time with his buddies this month. He's just finished his suspension from school and the grounding that Joel and I imposed for weekend activities, except for skiing. We felt that Jonathan needed some release. He's been working hard with his tutor to keep up with his studies.

Still, the tension in our house runs high and there are many silent moments.

After I drop the boys off at the bus and head home, the sky lightens to a silvery sheen. Lingering a moment on the steps before going back inside the house, I absorb the quiet, the stillness. The snow is crisp underfoot and the air is clear. It would be so nice to take a long walk with Joel today like we used to. Guiltily, I swallow this simple desire, my wish melting to fantasy as quickly as the snowflakes melt on my cheeks. I go inside and lock the door.

Upstairs, from Daniel's room, Joel calls me to join him. His face is beaming with pleasure.

"When I took Daniel to the bathroom this morning, his diaper was completely dry."

I smile too, glad to celebrate my son's success.

It would be nice to remain in this frame of mind, but my emotions jerk up and down so rapidly. We were expecting an attendant to arrive at noon today to look after Daniel so we could go to the luncheon reception of a friend's daughter's bat mitzvah. As eager to leave as Jonathan was this morning, I stand at the front door peering between the curtains, listening for the sound of a car engine.

The numbers on my watch keep advancing: 12:10 p.m., 12:20 p.m., 12:30 p.m. The attendant doesn't show. A call to the agency provides no explanation or offer of a substitute. In frustration, I slam down the receiver, ready to exchange my dressy suit for a pair of jeans. Instead, I call my brother Yaron and am relieved that he and Sue can spell us for a few hours. With a wave of appreciation, we leave the house a little after 1:00 p.m. and arrive at the reception, finding the guests still mingling over hors d'oeuvres. We greet our hosts, wish them a *Mazel Tov* and begin to socialize.

The dinging of a fork against crystal invites us all to be seated. In between the soup and salad courses, there are some speeches, and then a special singing performance by the bat mitzvah girl, whose voice is lovely. Joel checks his watch and gently taps my thigh. Our time is up. We must leave now before the main course is even served. I feel like Cinderella, whose coach is about to be converted to a pumpkin, her fancy gown back to rags. Quietly we slip away.

That night, I have a hard time falling asleep, turning from one side to the other to get comfortable. I fluff up the pillow; then add another. No, too high. Meanwhile, beside me, my husband sleeps soundly, his knees bumping mine. As I turn over, he flings an arm around me, a heavy weight encircling my waist. I wriggle to the far side of the bed, listening to the dull drone of the intercom connected to my son's room. Daniel is asleep. We've put his mattress on the floor and buttressed it with pillows in case he should roll off instead of renting a hospital bed with adjustable sidebars. We want his room to be as normal as possible.

When I drift to sleep, visions of my older son fill my dreams. He's speeding down a ski slope, charging across the ice, or water-skiing behind the boat, his hair pulled back in a ponytail that's bobbing in the wind. I picture him sprawled on his bed doing his homework or crouched on the carpet in the basement with his eyes glued to the TV screen for his favourite SEGA hockey game. Now there he is, peacefully dozing on a sun-drenched beach before dashing off to further action. With horror, I watch as the sand dunes slowly transform into crisp white linens, the bright rays of the sun into glaring fluorescent lights. Beeps and buzzing machines displace the roar of motorboats. I jerk and shake, forcing myself awake, as if to adjust the tracking on my internal video.

He's home now, I remind myself, gratefully. Asleep in his own room, just down the hall.

On Sunday morning, I awaken early. Hyper-alert to the sounds of the intercom, I haven't slept well. I'll get used to this, I think, as I carry the intercom unit around with me, plugging it into the kitchen first and then into the laundry room. There are extra tasks to do — thickening Daniel's drinks with a special gel that sets the liquid, loading additional laundry because of his incontinence. Wherever I am, I listen for him.

The day is busy. Joel helps Daniel shower and sits with him at meals. We take turns playing games with him. Several of his friends drop by, and although excited by their visits, our son is exhausted by 4:00 p.m.

"He needs to nap, Joel. Why don't we take him back to Hugh

Mac now and go out to a movie? Jonathan has plans with some friends to watch a sports program and it'd be nice to have a break together."

The movie accomplishes what it's meant to, taking our minds off our worries. At home, the light on the answering machine is flashing with a single message. Probably my mother, I think, as I press the button to retrieve the message. An unfamiliar voice identifies herself as the night nurse at Hugh Mac.

"I want to assure you that your son is now fine, but he fell out of his wheelchair. I found him lying on the floor with the urinal bottle beside him. Once again, rest assured that he wasn't hurt."

My husband erupts in anger. "How could they allow this to happen? Where was the supervision? We can't be with him twenty-four hours a day."

I'm upset, too. If this is the price to pay for my pleasure, it doesn't seem fair. Slowly we calm down, and as our anger dissolves, we're left with feelings of helplessness. Our son is so vulnerable. As he asserts his independence while his judgement is still impaired, there are bound to be problems. Although nothing serious happened this time, it could.

Sometimes, I wish it were like buying a car where you can go in and choose from the available options. New and improved, like the advertisements suggest. But we're not buying a new model and we have no choice in the deficits Daniel will have. Potentially paralysed vocal cords. A non-functional right arm. Inability to walk. Impairments in short-term memory and judgement. We don't want any of these for our son.

I write a draft of a newsletter, including some of these thoughts. Unsure whether to send it because the emotions expressed are so raw, I show it to two friends. Gerri tells me it's a privilege to have such thoughts shared with her. Ellen says that it sounds like I'm looking for pity, that I'm trying to make others feel bad because I'm hurting. Her comments distress me because they ring true. I'm tired of people offering me their platitudes, telling me how much they admire my strength. Sometimes, I want them to see my pain, too. However, Joel agrees with Ellen. People just want to hear the good parts about Daniel's progress, to be encouraged, not depressed. So I revise my fifth newsletter and send it off.

February 1, 1994
Dear Family and Friends,

Daniel transferred to Hugh MacMillan Rehabilitation Centre almost three weeks ago and it's been a very positive move. He's actively involved in all kinds of therapy, in the resource room with the special education teacher, and in recreational activities. The philosophy of Hugh Mac is to involve the family as much as they wish to be, but we have purposely stayed away during the day to allow the therapists an opportunity to get to know Daniel and work on their assessments of him. So far we've been getting snippets of information as feedback. We're invited to follow him through his activities throughout a full morning and will do that on Friday. A full team assessment report will occur at week six.

The big issue has been his level of fatigue. The staff members are very flexible and try to adjust the individualized schedule to meet his needs, but he's required an unusual number of rest periods. The doctor decided on Wednesday to cut back on some of his medications to see if that would make a difference, and already some improvement has been noted.

When we took Daniel back to Hugh Mac after his first weekend home, he joined a recreational therapist while we chatted to one of the nurses. Then two of his friends dropped in and we walked them down to the activity centre to find him. Daniel wasn't there. Instead, he was in the gym with two plastic hockey sticks and a basketball on his wheelchair tray. The therapist was setting up a hockey net and Daniel had a big grin on his face. The therapist outfitted his friends with wheelchairs to join him in a game of wheelchair hockey. Jonathan found the experience comforting and we were much more content leaving Daniel here than at Sunnybrook.

The personalized care and attention that our son is receiving at Hugh Mac is just what we wanted, so Joel and I were surprised to find ourselves feeling so low. In part, I think we were suffering withdrawal symptoms. We had been so intensely involved with him, especially during the last three weeks of his stay at Sunnybrook, that limiting our visiting time has been an adjustment. Then in contrast, we've started taking him home for the whole weekend, so we are intensely involved for that forty-eight- to fifty-hour period with little respite.

Jonathan's explanation probably comes closest to explaining our feelings. At Sunnybrook, the patients on the C5 ward were quite severely disabled, and his brother looked good in comparison after he began showing progress. Now Daniel is the most needy patient on the head injury unit at Hugh Mac. The residents who were not discharged at Christmas are well on the road to recovery. Granted, we don't know what these adolescents looked like when they first arrived. Besides, we should be hopeful for the gains that we know Daniel will make. Unfortunately, rational reasoning just seems to get in the way of our emotions.

There are numerous signs that our son is slowly improving. His trunk control is much greater and he's much more mobile in his wheelchair, manoeuvring with his left foot around the rooms and through the hall. The physiotherapy focus so far has been to teach him independent transfers to and from his wheelchair while under supervision. His muscles, particularly on the left side, are redeveloping their former strength.

The occupational therapist comes in early two mornings a week to work on ADL (activities of daily living): dressing, shaving, and personal care routines. The other days, nursing staff supervise these activities. Functional skills and independent performance are emphasized and there is always a cognitive and memory component to each skill.

Daniel still has no voice, but his language skills are increasing. His whispering is most effective after a nap when he's still lying down; otherwise, we're into lip reading. His vocabulary and ability to exchange ideas are greater. He has a graphic output device on loan from the Augmentative Communication Service to help with writing when oral communication skills break down.

He's showing more initiative, as well as becoming much more assertive and much harder to distract when he gets an idea fixed in his mind. On Sunday, he insisted on calling his friends earlier in the morning than I thought advisable and assured me that they would be awake. Now his friends leave wake-up times of 11:00 a.m. or 12:00 p.m. beside their numbers to avoid those 9:30 a.m. calls.

Yesterday, Joel visited after Daniel's nap and asked him if he remembered being home on the weekend.

Daniel said, "Yes, I love to be home."

"We love to have you home," Joel replied.

"Then why do you keep sending me away?" he asked sadly.

Joel explained that he needed the people at Hugh Mac to help him get better and do all the things that he wanted to do.

"You can do it!" Daniel said.

"But I don't know how," Joel answered. "The people here went to school for four years to study how to do it and I didn't."

"You and Mom can learn quickly," Daniel said.

While this exchange instils a touch of sadness in us, it also provides a measure of hope as Daniel is showing more cognitive awareness.

Love,

Lainie

CHAPTER TWENTY-FIVE

Although I no longer have to deliver a stimulation program to Daniel, my afternoons are crowded with medical and therapeutic appointments. One day, during a speech therapy session, I watch my son trying to blow bubbles through a straw into a jar of liquid. It reminds me of the times my brothers and I would play with our milk instead of drinking it. We loved those frothy bubbles that floated up the sides of the glass. Sometimes, if we were lucky, a big bubble would encase the rim like a dome, sealing the glass completely — so tempting for a small finger to pop.

Daniel doesn't look like he's having any fun.

"In order to keep the liquid up, his palate must activate," the speech therapist says. "It's working a little, but not under voluntary control. Air is still going out his nose."

She demonstrates by holding a small mirror under his nostrils. The mirror quickly fogs.

"Let's take a break, Daniel. We can see you're working hard. We'll practise more next time."

Friday, when Joel and I meet with the medical director of the rehab centre, he uses a model of the brain to explain the effects of Daniel's injury, and I jot down notes.

"The velocity of the impact sent shock waves through the brain, causing shearing, tearing, and recoil. In addition to the large haematoma that, as you know, was evacuated from the left side of his brain, it's likely that there are many microscopic subcortical haemorrhages in the grey matter, thereby creating a diffuse" — I knew he meant widespread — "effect in his closed head injury, rather than just a focal or localized effect. There's also evidence of intraventricular blood on the right side of the brain that could be a result of tearing of vessels or from the initial haematoma itself."

We nod at the doctor, suggesting we understand. What's becoming clear to me is the severity of my son's injury — how close to death he was when the paramedics in the ambulance got to the accident site. We've learned that his score was three on the Glasgow Coma Scale that ranges from three to fifteen. Less than twenty years ago, the most advanced neurosurgery techniques couldn't have saved my son. But is modern medicine kinder? The research still suggests poor outcome results for those whose GCS scores are less than eight. Severely brain injured — that's Daniel's category!

When I lie in bed at night, reading the latest research from the journals I've borrowed from the Brain Injury Association library, I no longer share the information I'm learning with my husband. What's the use in telling him that our son is likely to have lifelong problems with locomotion, social interactions, communication, and problem-solving skills? Joel can't bear to hear the statistics: eighty per cent of those who sustain such a catastrophic injury don't return to school or work. It doesn't help me to learn this, either. My husband is determined that Daniel will fall into the other category — the twenty per cent who do succeed. So I'm trying to focus on those articles that discuss effective techniques for rehabilitation.

Pointing to a different section of the brain, the doctor continues his explanation. "Daniel's fatigue and difficulty with endurance may be related to damage in the brain stem. We'll wait and see if the neurosurgeon feels an MRI would be helpful, although this test is just a picture that doesn't predict function. Structure versus function, that's the question. In the meantime, I'm going to try reducing his medications and see if that makes a difference."

"What about vocalizing?" I ask.

"Whispering is a specific vocal cord set that doesn't involve movement. We don't know if there's been nerve damage to his vocal cords caused by the injury itself or during intubation. We do know the brain can regrow fibres and form new connections. However, it can't regrow nerve cells."

As I try to digest this information, he says, "I'd like to refer him for a fibre optic assessment of the vocal chords to evaluate structure and movement. My secretary will let you know when the appointment's arranged."

Joel emerges from the office silently. His hands are curled into soft fists, his shoulders hunched, his eyes downcast. He looks like a defeated boxer leaving the ring, although his wounds aren't visible. I don't say anything. By now, I know it will take him at least a day to recuperate. Then he'll plunge back into action. By sheer dint of will, he's determined to make a difference in our son's outcome. This faith, this single-minded purpose, is all that sustains him.

CHAPTER TWENTY-SIX

How far removed this therapy room is from the gymnastics class that Daniel took so long ago. It's February, and the bars here are spaced wheelchair-width apart. The physiotherapist locks the wheelchair wheels and helps Daniel stand, holding him steady as he reaches out his left hand to grasp the bar. His right arm is clenched in a V, his fist curled tightly against his chest. Too much tone, they tell us. His muscles are tight when he needs them to be relaxed, and they resist straightening.

My eyes remain glued on Daniel, following his moves like they used to during his gymnastics class. He was about five then, a young boy in red shorts. Behind the mirrored wall, we mothers sat, some chatting, others knitting or reading a book or magazine, glad of the respite from front-line duty, looking up now and then to take a glance at their kids. But I enjoyed watching him, my little boy in red shorts. Short, sturdy, not quite stocky, with his shock of brown hair and an intense look of concentration that was broken by broad grins with each successful flip. Steady arms firmly grasped metal bars as taut legs plunged through. Such graceful movement.

Today he wobbles, leaning to the left.

"That's it, Daniel. Look straight ahead. Lift your head. Now bend your knee and lift your right foot."

Slowly, deliberately, he bends his right knee. His toes catch against the floor as if he's trying to kick a soccer ball. They stick. Behind him, an assistant bends to lift his right foot and move it forward.

Like a drunk who's misplaced the curb, Daniel lurches. His left hand grips the bar, his knuckles whitening as the skin pulls taut. He grimaces.

"Well done. Now lean on your right leg. Don't worry. I'm holding you. Take a step with your left."

His forehead wrinkles while his chest heaves up and down like the ocean's waves. Bending his knee, he raises it up and strikes his heel, then toes on the ground.

A real step!

Bursting into a grin, his face tells us: See, I'm walking, just like I knew I would.

The exercises are monotonous, constant repetitive movements to improve trunk control and balance. Daniel lies on a mat. He can roll onto his side now, but bends his knees slowly. Pressing his left arm onto the mat, he tries to raise himself upright. In kinesiology, the study of movement, students learn that it takes ten thousand repetitions to learn a new motor skill. I wonder if it takes the same number to relearn one? Last summer, when Joel and I started golf lessons, there were so many pieces of information to absorb: the grip, stance, ball position, and weight transfer. Too much all at once and I found it so frustrating that I could barely hit the ball.

How do you bypass the thought process and turn the activity into automatic motion? I think about the time I learned to ride a bike, my father helping me balance, making sure my feet were positioned securely on the pedals and then running behind me down the sidewalk, his hand gripping the back seat to steady me. How many trials did it take for him to feel confident enough to let go? For me to take off on my own? At first, I was so conscious of gripping the handlebars, pedalling furiously, and trying to stay upright. So many things to remember.

When Alyssa was six, Joel taught her to ride a bike the same way I learned. Daniel was different. When he was only four and a half, Joel was planning to attach training wheels to his sister's outgrown two-wheeler for him. But Alyssa suggested that he try it without them.

"Let's go to the park," she said. "I bet he can do it on the grass."
And he did, the very first time.

This new stage of Daniel's therapy makes me think of childhood, motion, and learning — spontaneous learning. In the same way we didn't need to teach Daniel how to ride a bike, parents don't teach kids how to walk. We wait, sometimes impatiently, then eagerly applaud that first tentative step. Hovering nearby, we anticipate the inevitable fall. But baby legs are sturdy and baby bums well padded. It's easier with no pride involved. The next step will soon be taken and we'll have a little one toddling, and then before long, running around the house.

Now the learning isn't that easy. In physical therapy, each movement is calculated, premeditated, controlled. Directing each action, the therapist tries to re-build what was previously performed automatically. With Daniel, the pace is sluggish. He's so different now.

As a young mother it would take me so long to get Daniel bundled up in a snowsuit with his hat, mittens, and boots. A squirming toddler, he wouldn't lie still on the floor no matter what the impending reward — a ride in a toboggan, the stroller, or car.

Now everything about him is slow. Time stretches out as if you're gazing at an unending forest with trees so thick you can't see the light shining through. At times, I'd like to speed things up, do things for him. Sometimes I have to. I put on his jacket, do up his zipper, bend over to put on his shoes and lace them. Then immediately I'm sorry, wishing I didn't have to do these things at all. On weekends, I watch his deliberate movements as he dresses himself, lying on his back so he won't lose his balance. He lifts his buttocks to pull on his sweatpants and struggles to bend his right knee to get on his sock. If he gets his head stuck in his shirt, one of us has to be nearby to straighten things out.

This morning after his shower, he lies on our carpet putting on his clothes when he has a bout of bowel incontinence. His face crumples up like a piece of paper wadded and tossed in a garbage can, as close to crying as we've seen, but stopped somehow, before the tears actually start.

"Mess. Carpet," he whispers to Alyssa.

"Don't worry, we'll clean it up," she whispers back.

For now, the morning's embarrassing episode is forgotten, at least pushed aside, while his dripping wet grin emerges from the swimming pool. He's just put his face underwater and held his breath, blowing bubbles to the count of ten. The longest time yet. Joel, Alyssa, and I are with him, cheering him on.

The Hugh Mac pool is a feast of visual stimulation; the walls painted with colourful murals of sea creatures cavorting underwater, and overhead, bright kites with long streaming tails float like fanciful birds against a rich blue sky. A warm place with friendly faces. Young staff with welcoming smiles, not the bored, disdainful expressions of lifeguards showing off their tanned pecs and rippling abs at a public beach or community pool. Joel transfers Daniel from his wheelchair to a swim chair, a special seat that can be wheeled directly into the water. Now that Daniel is learning to balance upright, there's no need for the Hoyer Lift that was used in the hospital to transfer him in and out of bed.

The pool is crowded on Saturdays, especially this hour for community swim. Children squeal and splash in the shallow end, towed on inflatable floats by parents who stop to chat to one another and catch up on the week's news. An older woman, stiff with arthritis, makes her way slowly down the ramp. Released into the water, she lays back, her head tilted upwards to keep the petals on her bathing cap dry. In the deep end are the more serious swimmers, but even they don't race back and forth or jackknife at the wall to flip around underwater like the hard-core swimmers at the Y or high school pools. This water is warm, almost bathlike. Too warm for speed.

With just his bathing suit on, the asymmetry in Daniel's body is obvious. His right shoulder, arm, and leg muscles have atrophied, producing a slack and skinny look, while his left side has regained some of its former strength. How strange to see half of him as slender as Joel who wheels Daniel slowly into the water. When the water is about waist deep, Daniel stands, grabbing onto the ledge for a moment. A few weeks ago, when Joel began taking him to the pool, Daniel would cautiously let go of the ledge and try to balance, clutching his father's hands. Now he clasps his left hand onto Joel's right wrist and takes a few tentative steps, then a few more. Soon he is walking across the width of the pool. It's amazing to see him walk in water, something he still can't accomplish on land. The buoyancy of the water helps.

At the far side of the pool, he grasps the ledge and takes a rest. A young man with a life jacket on comes over to talk to him. He introduces himself and tells us his story.

"Two years ago, I was thrown from a horse and broke my neck. Paralysed from the neck down, I spent almost a year in the hospital. The doctors told me I'd never walk again, but look at me. I'm walking. I never gave up."

"Me too," Daniel mouths.

Encouraged by Tom's story, Daniel decides to swim, not only on his back, but on his front too. Holding his breath, my son moves his left arm up and over in a front-crawl stroke, displacing the water as he pulls it through. His right elbow sticks up at an awkward angle, a shark's fin, immobile. But both his legs are flutter kicking — his right one too.

The chill of the air surprises us when we come out of the water. Alyssa scurries, shivering, right into the change room. Wrapping a towel around my shoulders, I wait for Joel to push Daniel up the ramp, bundle up both my guys in towels, and then head to the showers myself. Alyssa and I stand there talking, recapping the achievements we've just witnessed, while the hot water cascades over us. There's no need to rush. We'll have plenty of time to dry our hair. We know it will be a long wait until Daniel is ready.

The next day, Daniel decides he wants to write a letter to his friend, Rachel, in Switzerland, so I set him up on the computer in my home office. Using his left index finger, he hunts and pecks for letters, finally typing out a sentence: I want to go skiing to beautiful your body.

I wonder what he means. Last March, when we were skiing at Whistler Mountain, Rachel's visit overlapped with ours for a few days. I remember she and Daniel skied together one day, and sometimes hung out in the late afternoons, strolling through the village or watching videos with Jonathan in our hotel suite. Rachel even got Daniel to try line dancing with her one evening. The following after-noon, when she demonstrated some of the moves they had learned, he seemed uncomfortable that she'd share any of this with us. At seventeen, he usually wanted to keep his friends and activities private.

Now, as I stand behind my son, I help him adjust what he's written. Then I sit down on the couch and wait for him to call me again. This time the sentence is so incoherent that I can't get it to make sense, despite several tries. Disappointed and frustrated, I leave the room and lumber down the hall to my bedroom, where Joel and Alyssa have been lounging and chatting.

"Where's my patience?" I ask, as if expecting someone to look under the bed and find it. "I used to be a good teacher. All those years working with students with learning disabilities. Why can't I help my own son?"

"It's okay, Mom," Alyssa says. "I'll take over."

My husband beckons me to lie down beside him. As I cuddle into his arms, he strokes my back, reassuring me that all will be fine. I bury my head in his shoulder and try to relax under the steady touch of his hand. A few minutes later, we hear our daughter's voice emit a strangled cry. Rushing into my office, Joel and I see Daniel sitting impassively at the computer, oblivious to his sister's distress.

"What's wrong?" I ask.

Alyssa just stands there, covering her mouth with her hands to stifle her sobs. Joel hugs her while I read what's on the computer screen: "I very scared to tell you how sad I am, but I okay."

I burst into tears, too.

It feels like a punch in my gut, this first direct exposure to Daniel's feelings. How can he move so quickly from such raw emotions to neatly wrapping things up? It's like approaching a chasm filled with sadness and then backing away, knowing the gap's too wide to bridge, the descent too scary.

Sniffling into a tissue, Alyssa pulls herself back together and hugs her brother.

"You're right, Daniel. You're okay."

"You're definitely okay," Joel says.

I print the letter, but never mail it to Rachel.

CHAPTER TWENTY-SEVEN

Valentine's Day: my father's birthday. This year feels like a bittersweet celebration as we mark his eightieth year. In the past, we would all gather at my home for dinner or go out to a restaurant together. It's now gotten too hard to transport him away from the veteran's nursing home where he lives, yet my mother is anxious to mark this day in some special way. She has arranged a party, a simple celebration with family members augmented by a few friends, including some other ailing residents of K-wing and their wives.

The venue for the party turns out to be better than we had hoped. The cafeteria in K-wing is festooned for Valentine's Day with balloons, red and white streamers, paper Cupids, and crimson hearts. We have a section cordoned off for our use and it looks festive. My father assumes that we've decorated the room just for him and seems delighted that we've gone to such effort.

Dad looks good today, dressed in a white shirt, tie, and sweater instead of the sweatsuit that has become his standard garb. My mother is buoyant, acting the role of hostess, making sure that all guests are comfortably settled around the long table that's laden with fruit platters and an array of cakes.

The K-wing wives talk of the entertainer who is due to perform in the lounge later that day. "Such a good pianist," one says. "Plays all the hits from the forties. Even gets some of these old soldiers singing along." I find that hard to believe as I watch their husbands, whose lolling heads droop against their wheelchair headrests. I've never heard any of them talk.

We're pleased that despite his advancing memory problems, Dad still recognizes everyone and greets them warmly. That is, everyone but Daniel.

He points to the young man sitting silently in the wheelchair near the end of the table near him and asks, "Who is he? And why doesn't he say anything?"

"It's Daniel, your grandson," I reply.

"Well, whoever he is, you'd better give him a piece of birthday cake. He looks like he needs it."

CHAPTER TWENTY-EIGHT

It's *Reading Week* in *late February and many of Daniel's* friends are back in town from university. On Friday, Alana and Sari come to the rehab centre and watch him in a physiotherapy session. I'm there too, because he's scheduled to be measured for a new wheelchair today, a customized model that the staff have recommended we purchase. It seems like such a commitment, but they tell us that there's no point in just renting one as we've been doing for the past month. Even if Daniel learns to walk, he'll need it for distances, they say, for outings to the zoo, the Science Centre, Canada's Wonderland, and museums. I can't even imagine my son wanting to go to any of these places with his friends. Are his interests supposed to change now that he has had a brain injury?

The physiotherapist helps Daniel walk down the hall with a walker and then secures him on the exercise bike, strapping his right foot onto the pedal. He pedals energetically, smiling at his friends. With the girls watching, he seems to be working even harder than usual.

That night his friends, Jodi and Jaimie, join us for *Shabbat* dinner, while on Sunday Phil and four other camp friends come over for brunch. Even Rachel's here, visiting from Switzerland. The whole house is hopping, with Alyssa home for the week and her friends dropping in too. There's laughter that ranges from tinny chuckles to loud deep guffaws — sounds I've been missing. I don't mind the extra time spent in the kitchen; it feels quite festive with so many young people around.

The week seems to race by. Our evenings are filled with the standard activities, although it's different with Daniel's friends around. Their support and encouragement energize him, and the rest of us too. On Monday evening, Jodi joins the regulars at the Hugh Mac pool and I come along, equipped with a video camera to tape the action. The guys are zany. Whooping and hooting like little kids, they surround themselves with balls and hoops, encouraging Daniel to join in the fun. With Joel behind him, ready to catch him should he lose his balance, Daniel tries to lob a ball into the hoop net guarded by Andrew. His aim is way off.

"And Daniel has the puck. No, he's passed it back to Jaimie. Now it's Jaimie, sneaking up the sideboards and stick handling that puck. Whew, that's close. A wonderful save by our goalie," reports Andrew, with the breathless excitement of a sportscaster.

I laugh, jiggling the camera, as Matt sneaks up from behind and dunks Andrew underwater. Spewing bubbles like a whale through its blowhole, Andrew swims through the centre of the hoop and swoops it much closer to Daniel. This time when my son throws the ball, it lands right in the middle of the hoop.

"Well, folks. What did I tell you? You gotta keep your eye on this young man. He's definitely going places."

The next night, Jodi and Jaimie offer to join us at Variety Village. I wish they could come with us, but there's no room on the special bus that Daniel and I ride with the other Hugh Mac participants. They arrange to meet us there.

The recreational therapists are efficient, checking names off the list and directing the flow of traffic. Still, it takes a while for everyone to get loaded onto the bus and strapped into place. I find myself seated near the back beside another mother I haven't met before, a young woman with deep blue eyes and a nervous laugh. She introduces me to her seven-year-old daughter, who was hit by a car a month ago while riding her bike. She's a pretty blonde girl with a leg brace and a patch over one eye. Her mother has moved to Toronto, leaving her two younger children at home with her husband and his mother, who's helping out.

"I'm hoping we'll get to go home in two more weeks. That will be good, to be home again." Then her voice fades to a whisper, "But she's so needy and the little ones won't understand. How can I take care of them all?"

I don't answer. I think of my youngest child. Am I taking care of him? It feels that most of the time I'm telling Jonathan to do some-thing, "Please, set the table. Take out the garbage. If your homework's done, why don't you play a game with your brother?"

When Reading Week ends and everyone leaves, it's hard to return to the status quo of just Joel, Jonathan, and myself. The sudden quiet in the house seems deafening.

CHAPTER TWENTY-NINE

We've been invited to Phoenix to attend the bar mitzvah of my cousin's son, Ryan. The timing seems ideal, coinciding with March break when I'll be off work. For a few days I consider the feasibility of taking Daniel to the celebration. Thinking about other family gatherings, I picture us being embraced by my aunts, uncles, and cousins, buoyed with their good wishes and love, enlivened by the younger children. I block out the reality of the difficulties of travel, Daniel's special needs for food, the care and supervision he requires. Then I talk to Bob, the social worker at Hugh Mac. Diplomatically, he helps me realize how farfetched this fantasy is.

Daniel is suffering from neurofatigue, a condition that often follows brain trauma: the brain goes into shutdown mode when it's overloaded. The brain has no second wind to recoup energy, unlike a marathon athlete who can keep on going even when exhausted. We've watched Daniel simply fade, collapse into sleep, and take hours to recover. This trip is too ambitious an undertaking, but I don't want to go without him. He always looks forward to coming home on weekends, so we're not prepared to leave him. Bob encourages us to consider alternatives.

"Why not take Jonathan away for a few days midweek? You know that Daniel will be well cared for here."

On the Monday of March break we find ourselves in a bus driven on the left side of the road. We're in Nassau, and we've chosen a hotel away from the bustle of the casinos and big city life. The bus passes through a small town with a central square of interlocking red bricks, continuing onward past gated mansions with lush vegetation on one side of the road. On the other side are small shacks with barefoot children playing in the yards.

Arriving at the hotel, we find we're staying in a small villa, divided into four apartments. An elaborately carved highboy is the focal piece of furniture, brightly patterned rugs cover the shiny parquet floor, a large ceiling fan hums overhead, and tall wooden shutters open to expose the sliding door to a private patio. Just beyond is the ocean. When we step outside, we're surrounded by eternal elements: sand, water, sun, and sky.

What more could we want? It seems perfect, but without Daniel and Alyssa, there's a sense of looming emptiness. Our beach holidays have always included the five of us, often with other families and their children too, providing built-in companionship and as much activity as anyone wanted. Swimming, snorkelling, tennis, beach volleyball. There was always someone who had a new suggestion to make. Let's paint ceramics, visit the local market, or take a jet ski tour to a coral reef. Who wants to rent a boat for deep-sea fishing or go horseback riding? Not today, thanks. I'll just walk on the beach and relax under a thatched umbrella, reading undisturbed for hours on end while digging my toes in the sand.

Joel and I have agreed to a moratorium about discussing Daniel, and over the next few days we find ourselves silenced unnaturally. For months now, that's been the mainstay of our conversation. Gone are the days when we would go for evening walks with the dog after dinner and talk about the kids or work. I usually told anecdotes of things that had happened or ideas I had read that day, while Joel liked to talk about his projects, his visions for expanding his firm's practice in innovative ways. I miss these talks and we can't recapture them. People don't understand about the all-consuming nature of this trauma. Most other topics seem trivial. It's so hard to find pleasure, even in this lovely tropical setting.

The sun shines and the waves crest, inviting us into the ocean, yet Joel prefers to sit by himself in the shade of the patio. To compensate, I try to engage Jonathan, offering to swim with him, play cards, or rent a double kayak. There aren't many teenagers at this resort, at least none close to his age, so he tags along with me reluctantly. Sometimes in the mornings or late afternoons, the three of us make our way to the driving range and practise hitting golf balls. We can't work up the energy to actually play a game. Besides, Jonathan and I aren't good enough anyway.

On Friday, there's almost a sense of relief when we pack our bags and board the shuttle to the airport to return home.

My mother returns in pain from the bar mitzvah in Phoenix. Try as she might, she can't hide it. Spasms in her leg radiate in shooting stabs, making her grimace and clench her teeth. She tries to pretend it doesn't matter, but sometimes her leg buckles out beneath her when she stands, causing her to lose her balance.

"It's a problem with your spine," the doctor says. "I'm hoping it will repair itself within three months. Otherwise we'll need to operate."

"But I'm seventy-five years old already."

"Right, and you don't want to live like this, do you? Curtailing all your activities. You can't even drive anymore. You're not living alone, are you?"

"Of course I am. And you'd better not suggest I move in with my children. They've already asked me and there's no way I'm going to be a burden on them. I'm perfectly capable of taking care of myself."

Shrugging his shoulders, the doctor looks at me. What a feisty lady. Her spirits are still strong, although for the moment her body is betraying her.

After the appointment, she slowly makes her way back down the hall to the hospital entrance, leaning heavily on the cane I've insisted she use. Briefly we argue, and I convince her to wait while I get the car from the parking lot. Exiting through the revolving doors, I glance back to ensure she's seated. I'm struck by how frail she looks, her sturdy bulk softened like ice cream left out too long on the counter. When I was growing up, my mother always seemed so strong. Her wide fingers never struggled to open jars, and her thumb was so thick it couldn't fit into the hole of a standard bowling ball when we played tenpins on Sunday afternoons. She and my father played in a couples' league and they both had customized balls. I liked to watch her stride down the lane and fling out that ball. Smash, the pins would flail, as if cowering in fear. Strike! She was one of the top scorers in the women's division, with a shelf full of trophies.

On the drive home, I stop to pick up fresh produce, bread, and some prepared food so she won't have to cook. I carry the groceries into her apartment, but she won't let me help her put them away.

"I'm fine. Just fine," she says, shooing me away like she would a stray cat.

"I'll phone you tomorrow and if you need anything, anything at all, please call. Okay?" I say.

After dinner, when Alyssa phones for her nightly check-in, her voice sounds strained.

"Mom, when I was walking out of the Economics class today, my legs suddenly buckled. I was heading to the elevator, but they couldn't hold me up. It was as if they didn't even belong to me."

"Are you all right?"

"No. Two of my classmates found me collapsed in a heap in the hallway. I couldn't get up. I just couldn't stand up. They lifted me and practically carried me to the elevator, then one of them drove me home in my car. Mom, I'm in such pain. What should I do?"

I'm ready to jump in my car and rush to her side. I picture myself holding my little girl on my lap, rocking her, cooing and telling her that soon she'll be better. Where are those sturdy limbs that used to run and jump, turn cartwheels, dance, and ski down the mountains? It's hard enough to witness my mother hurting, but for several years now, we've watched our daughter live with recurring pain — in her knees, hips, and shoulders. None of the medical tests have been conclusive. Perhaps rheumatoid arthritis, but not likely, some say. Joint problems, connective tissue. The doctors can't agree. Still, we're relieved to learn that the condition isn't life threatening. But she wants some answers. What am I supposed to say to her? About any of this?

There's so much happening in my life right now, so many stressors — Daniel's neurofatigue and slow recuperation, my father's deterioration, Jonathan's sullenness, my mother in pain, and now my daughter too, with her flare-up. One of my colleagues at work joked that I must be living under a dark cloud. Don't get too close, she told me. The problems might spread and she didn't think she could handle them. Can I? I don't feel particularly stoic. There are days when everything just seems so unfair, so overwhelming.

"Alyssa, you'd better come home. Have a friend drive you to the train tonight. We'll pick you up."

"I can't, Mom. Exams start in a few weeks and the professors are reviewing material. I'll be home in a few days anyway for Passover. My roommate will drive me in."

"So how are you going to manage now?"

"Susan's gone to rent me a wheelchair. I guess I'll use that for a few days."

Another wheelchair in the family.

I pause, remembering Joel's advice to compartmentalize issues and deal with them one at a time like he does at work.

"I'll try to get you another doctor's appointment when you're in town. Your aunt Sue said she had connections at the hospital, a pain clinic, I think she mentioned. I'll call her. In the meantime, take care of yourself, cutie. I'll speak to you tomorrow."

That evening, I linger in my bath, imagining myself once again on a beach inhaling the salt spray in the air. The hard-packed sand feels solid beneath my feet and the gently lapping waves, like friendly children, invite me into the ocean to play. I stretch out on my back, my arms akimbo, absorbing the soothing that floating brings. The blueness of sky meets blue-green water with just a thin pencilled outline of horizon. The sun embraces me. In the distance, there are children's voices and high-pitched laughter. I close my eyes and drift in the water. Suddenly, I can hear my daughter's voice. A little girl calling, "Mommy, Mommy, I need you."

I must rush to her side. The waves feel stronger now, no longer kind. They crash at me, their white tops mocking my feeble progress. Close to shore, I plant my feet in shifting sand. Pulling waves break them apart. My balance falters and I'm dragged under. When I emerge, gritty sand clings to my hair.

I sit up, blinking my eyes.

The bath water has turned tepid and I feel quite chilled. Pulling out the plug, I stare as the water swirls down the drain.

CHAPTER THIRTY

The mahogany table with its thick pedestal base anchored my grandparents' home. Their dining room contrasted sharply with the sleek modern look of my childhood house. Unlike the fresh green wall-to-wall carpeting in our suburban bungalow, a frayed rug of indeterminate colours tried unsuccessfully to reach into the corners of that room. Light entered through two narrow windows and the wallpaper had a flecked dark blue pattern.

To the left of the dining room was the parlour. In one corner stood a tall brass reading lamp and an easy chair of matted gold velvet that had long ago lost its sheen. This was my grandfather's favourite spot. With a Yiddish newspaper spread open on his lap, he could monitor the pulse of the whole house as my cousins and I raced from parlour to kitchen and then up the stairs to the bedrooms, playing tag and hide-and-seek, using the table's pedestal as home base. The youngest one could always be found with a thumb in his mouth, hiding behind my grandpa's chair.

"Please be quiet, kids," I recall my mother saying. "I've just put the baby down to sleep. Why don't you go outside to play?"

From the kitchen, my grandmother replied: "Leona, let the *kinder* be. If the baby is tired, he'll sleep. If not, not. I raised six children in this house and it was never quiet here."

Sighing, my mother entered the kitchen as my cousin, Judy, and I settled down at the large upright piano just outside the kitchen door. My feet dangled off the piano bench, not reaching the floor, and the keys felt cool to my touch. Judy, five years older, was already an accomplished pianist, but all I knew how to play was "Chopsticks." Our repetitive refrain blended with the rhythmic chopping sounds emerging from the kitchen as my grandmother, mother, and aunts sliced vegetables and minced ground beef in a large wooden bowl, then teased out circles that would become savoury meatballs. Smells wafted through the open doorway — simmering chicken soup, frying onions, and the sweet smell of cinnamon and honey for the sticky dessert that ended our meal. The pungent odour of freshly grated horseradish made my mouth pucker in anticipation of its bitter taste.

That mahogany table stands burnished in my memory — my mother's whole family crowded around it, aunts and uncles with elbows touching, children squirming. I remember my grandmother covering her head with a white lace shawl before lighting the holiday candles that gleamed from the sideboard, giving the room a special glow.

Smiling, I unfurl crisp white tablecloths over my dining room table and the extension table that joins it in the middle. Together they form a letter T extending through the open French doors into the front hall. There'll be sixteen of us for dinner tonight. Alyssa is lying down now, but my mother-in-law will soon come downstairs and offer to help. She'll set the tables for me, laying out freshly polished silverware, the glass dishes that we'll use for the next eight days of Passover, bowls of salt water, and wine glasses that will balance precariously on saucers, one of them inevitably tipping sometime during the evening meal.

Yesterday, when I climbed on a stool in the kitchen to take down the *Haggadot* we'll read from tonight, I found three rumpled booklets at the bottom of the pile. Embellished with drawings of the ten plagues and Moses raising his staff to part the Red Sea, prayers, and children's songs, they evoke junior kindergarten performances with my boys wearing green frog-shaped hats and leaping around. I'm amazed to find myself singing snatches of a song. "One morning when Pharaoh awoke in his bed, there were frogs on his pillow and frogs on his head." It seems like just yesterday that I'd shake a finger, admonishing four-year-old Jonathan, "Frogs are not welcome on my bed. Please go down to the basement to do your jumping."

As I place the *Haggadot* on the serving cart in my dining room, a creased parchment bag pokes out. Wedged inside are a long grey-white feather and a wooden spoon. They haven't been used in years, but I still can't bring myself to throw them out, either. When I was a child, my parents followed the ritual of hiding ten cubes of bread around the house just before Passover started. My brothers and I scavenged to find them and swept up all the crumbs with the feather into the spoon. The next morning, we stood outside with my father while he burned the bread and recited a prayer, formalizing the start of the holiday that's observed with the eating of only unleavened products.

When I bring a box of matzo into the rehab centre for my son to eat during the holiday, his nurse asks me, "Does matzo have any laxative properties?"

"Oh, no," I answer. "It tends to be constipating."

"Well then, I don't think he should have any for breakfast. He really needs to eat a bran muffin each morning. Moving his bowels is important, you know."

Nodding reluctantly, I tell myself it's just not feasible to have Daniel observe a kosher Passover this year. Besides, it's not as if he'd really care. He was always questioning why I held onto traditions; my answers never seemed to satisfy him. Leaving the rehab unit, I comfort myself with the thought that at least he'll be home with us for the two evening *seders* and will be part of our family holiday photos.

At the head of the table is my brother, Yaron, who's leading our service this year, a position formerly held by my father. Jonathan, as the youngest child, has the traditional role of asking the four questions that begin with, "Why is this night different from all other nights?" The answer unfolds as we recite the story of Exodus. Yaron has added verses of poetry and special readings in English to encourage the few of us who cannot read Hebrew to participate.

I wonder whether Daniel is following any of this. In classes at the rehab centre, I've watched him struggle to read simple paragraphs. He'll skip words or lines and be unable to remember or understand what he's just read. Sitting beside him, at the foot of the extension table where there's more space for his wheelchair, Alyssa helps him turn the pages. When she completes her reading, it's his turn next. We're ready to skip him, but he picks up his book and holds it out in front of him. We wait, silencing the scraping of chairs and the rustling of pages.

What we hear is a muted whisper — the almost inaudible chant of Hebrew words strung together, flowing freely from some recess of his brain that holds this memory intact. Words of my father, my grandfather, our ancestors. The same words that are now being recited in Jewish homes across the globe. With napkins, we listeners dab our eyes, so astonished are we.

March 31, 1994
Dear Family and Friends,

Here's the latest info to answer your question, "How is Daniel doing?" He's continuing to make slow and steady progress. It's now seven months post-injury, and we're still waiting for him to regain his voice. The latest visit to the ENT (Ears, Nose, and Throat) clinic at Sunnybrook Hospital showed that there has been no physical damage to his vocal cords, so fortunately no surgery is required. We'll just have to wait for neurological recovery, for the brain's messages to connect to activate the vocal cords for speech.

Daniel's lack of voice does not prevent him from talking and we're beginning to see evidence of his former sense of humour. Today, a student nurse met Alyssa at the rehab centre. The nurse asked Daniel which one of them was older. He replied, "She's older, but I'm more mature!"

Physically, there's been improvement in the movement of his right leg. The physiotherapist and Joel use an electric stimulator to stimulate muscle contractions in his hamstring and we've noticed carry-over in muscle use. He's now able to bear weight when walking between parallel bars or when holding onto a railing. Joel installed thirty feet of railing in our basement to enable Daniel to practise at home and hung up mirrors on the end walls so he could watch himself and correct his posture. His progress has been encouraging.

The physiotherapist, Kim, is amazed by Daniel's performance in the gym. When she tries to have him do certain exercises in isolation, he isn't able to do so. However, when these exercises are incorporated into a sports format, the activity becomes automatic rather than requiring deliberate thinking. Just watch him lean to his right and maintain his trunk control while reaching for beanbags to throw through a basketball hoop and voila — success! His former athletic prowess is serving him well in his recovery.

He's also making good progress in his activities of daily living and is becoming much more independent. However, he still requires supervision for eating, dressing, bathing, and toileting. Because he still has restrictions on consumption of liquids, the nurses monitor all his eating and drinking. Daniel doesn't seem to appreciate their concerns, and the other day, he directed another patient to reach into a high cupboard for the cookies that he wanted. At least he's showing initiative.

Daniel is still affected by fatigue, which sometimes interferes with him keeping his prescribed schedule of therapy and which affects his power of attention and concentration. He was recently placed on a trial of Ritalin, a stimulant medication. It seems to be helping, but the results have to be formally analyzed. Everyone finds him more alert in the past few weeks. He has begun to socialize with his peers during lunchtime and in the evenings. The other day, when Dave, a fellow patient, was playing his guitar, Daniel accompanied him with a harmonica given to him by a friend. We didn't even know he knew how to play.

Daniel is kept very busy at Hugh Mac. He's involved in physiotherapy, speech therapy, occupational therapy, art therapy, and music therapy. In addition, there's a support group and cognitive retraining. He spends time each day in the resource room focussing on educational tasks. He's struggling to relearn basic computational skills. Reading and writing skills are also difficult for him. Further difficulties are evident in the language area: problems with word retrieval, associations, and categories. The progress in cognitive areas is not as readily noticeable to Daniel himself as his physical progress.

He's recently articulated a problem with double vision. If we come closer to him than eighteen inches, he announces that we are double. The solution has been to patch one of his eyes any time he reads or works on the computer. We're also waiting for an appointment with a neuro-ophthalmologist.

One of the activities that our son enjoys most is working out in the swimming pool at Hugh Mac, where three or four of his friends accompany him. Daniel is blessed by the active involvement of his many friends. They visit both at Hugh Mac and on the weekends at home. The professionals at Hugh Mac are flabbergasted by the dedication that these young adults show. His buddies are like a personal fan club, cheering him on and providing tremendous encouragement. Several of them also join Daniel's recreational group at Variety Village on Tuesday evenings that Daniel and I attend by special bussing.

Variety Village is a recreational complex for the physically disabled. Daniel works out in the weight room, stretching and strengthening his muscles. His left side has regained tremendous strength, which helps in his mobility. He also enjoys the group activities in the field house, a large gym area. He has participated in archery, floor hockey, and balloon badminton.

I'll keep you posted about further progress.

Love,

Lainie

CHAPTER THIRTY-ONE

My daughter has survived her April exams. Her professors were very accommodating and granted her special permission to write them while lying down in bed in her apartment. Now ensconced back in her own room, I can hear her bouncing on a big red therapy ball. Her legs are strapped with electrodes attached to a TENS unit that provides muscle stimulation, like the one Daniel uses to help him regain the use of his right leg. When Alyssa collapsed at university a few weeks ago, her muscles had already started to weaken. We're making the rounds of various medical specialists, but there's still no diagnosis or cure. With the guidance of a physiotherapist, she's trying to rebuild strength in her quads. She's anxious to regain mobility as quickly as possible because she has a summer job lined up with a downtown accountancy firm, one of her father's competitors.

While Daniel watches her exercise, Alyssa gives him pep talks.

"Daniel, I'm in a wheelchair too, and working to get out of it. Keep at your exercises. I know you'll do it."

I wish I shared her faith, her optimism. I believe in her recovery, but I'm not so sure about his. Some days, I question whether so much effort should be devoted to teaching Daniel to walk. Couldn't he live a reasonable life even if he were confined to a wheelchair? I'd rather see him regain some of the cognitive skills he's missing — not that we have a choice in the matter, since they're so much slower to recover.

The first time Joel and I visited the rehab centre, Bob, the social worker, took us on a tour. In the physiotherapy room, a teenage boy was strapped to a tilt table so he could experience the sensation of being upright. Eleven months post-injury and he was neither walking nor talking. Was this the prognosis for my son, too? When I expressed these fears to Joel, he looked at me quizzically. He hadn't made any association between the other teenager and our son. In his vision, Daniel would both walk and talk. There was no question in his mind.

I wonder whether I'm afraid to hold the same dreams as Joel, scared that they won't be realized. Perhaps I'm just being more realistic. We've both listened to the experts, but my beliefs are augmented by facts spouted in research texts, by speakers at the monthly meetings I've attended of the Brain Injury Association of Toronto, and by other parents I've spoken to. While most sources maintain the possibility of change, it's easy to read between the lines of what they're saying, "Slim chance. Don't reach for the stars."

One Friday evening as I'm preparing dinner, I watch Daniel sitting kitty-corner at the kitchen table across from my brother Amichai. My brother had offered to come to Canada from his home in Israel right after Daniel's injury, but there was really nothing he could do then to help. Now there is. For three weeks, he's looking after our mother, relieving me of the extra duties I'd assumed trying to take care of her. Despite her initial protests, she's delighted to have him here. She's still in pain and waiting for back surgery, but that's not likely to happen until June.

Amichai's dark hair with its hint of auburn is tied back in a ponytail, like Daniel used to wear. Between them lies a checkerboard. They gaze at it silently. When my son makes a move, my brother quickly responds, double jumping over Daniel's pieces.

"You're supposed to warn him," my mother says, lifting her head from the crossword puzzle she's been absorbed in. Her eyebrows pucker in disapproval.

"No, that's your job," Amichai replies. Plucking the discs from the board, he adds them to his growing pile.

Daniel isn't nearly as upset by his defeat as his grandmother. Nor am I. She'd like to coddle him, protect him from any further blows, but I'm delighted that he's been able to sustain his attention for so long. He still tires easily and it's hard for him to concentrate. Checkers is good training for him. There are so many skills involved: memory, visual scanning, curbing impulsivity, pre-planning. It doesn't really matter if he wins or loses.

Every afternoon at the rehab centre, a recreational therapist encourages the patients to get together in the solarium to play games or engage in arts and crafts. In this controlled environment, the teenagers practise appropriate social interactions: taking turns, talking politely to each other, sharing — skills they first learned in kindergarten and must now relearn. However, it's not unusual to find a board overturned or puzzle pieces swept to the floor. Low frustration tolerance is one of the hallmarks frequently shown following brain injury.

On Sunday morning, the doorbell rings. I reach for a dishtowel and head to the door, wiping my hands. There's another ring. A double staccato tone this time.

"Take it easy. I'm coming."

A stranger in shorts and sneakers stands on my porch. "Your husband needs you," she says.

I stare at her confusedly.

"Please," she points to the driveway. "He needs you now."

I race across the porch and down the stairs, the dishtowel swinging in my hand. I round the front of my daughter's car and gaze at the empty driveway.

"Joel? Joel?" My voice rises in pitch.

"We're here," he replies, his voice echoing from the embankment on the east side of the driveway.

The image that confronts me is an overturned wheelchair against a thick willow tree trunk. One wheel spins in slow rotation.

"Daniel!"

My head bobs around seeking my son. There he is, lying on the ground behind the tree, his head cradled in Joel's lap. I run down the hill and wrap my arms around both of them.

"Oh, God. What happened?" My voice, like an ill-tuned violin, screeches in high register.

"He's okay, I think," Joel says. "I'll tell you later. Put the wheelchair back together and help me transfer him to it."

I set the wheelchair upright, retrieve the seat from the grass and wrestle it back into place. Even empty, the wheelchair is hard to push across the lawn.

Joel raises Daniel to a seated position while I lock the wheelchair wheels in place. Blood drips from the corner of my son's mouth and skinny scratches streak across his forehead towards his left eye. He appears somewhat dazed and doesn't try to say anything.

My husband crouches behind him and wraps his arms around Daniel's chest. "Okay, you're going to stand up now. On three — here we go."

I lean forward to help Daniel balance as Joel pivots him in front of the wheelchair. Then Daniel eases himself back into the seat and his father buckles the safety straps.

Joel breathes heavily, taking in deep gulps of air. "I'll wait here a minute with him. Get some ice, okay?"

I race back up the slope and return quickly with a plastic bag filled with ice cubes and a damp towel that I use to wipe the blood off my son's mouth.

"He must have bitten his tongue," I say. "There's no cut on the outside."

Together we push the wheelchair over the grass, through the opening in the white wooden fence and back up the driveway to the house. Once we are settled back inside, Joel tells me the story.

"I needed to get my sunglasses from my car in the garage."

"So?" I ask, circling my hand to make him go faster.

"I had my back to him for only twenty or thirty seconds. During that time he unlocked the wheelchair brakes to move closer to Alyssa's car and unclicked his safety strap so he could look inside it."

"Why?"

"I don't know. When I turned around, he was gone. Careening down the embankment."

"He could have smashed his head on that tree," I say, picturing the spinning wheel of the wheelchair. It isn't hard to imagine a disaster scene. Fortunately, there doesn't appear to be anything really wrong — some scrapes on his chest and left hand, those few scratches on his face. The bleeding in his mouth has already stopped. We'll take him back to Hugh Mac to be checked out, just to be sure.

I breathe a sigh of relief. Secretly, I'm also relieved that I wasn't the one with Daniel when this happened. Not that Joel would blame me, but he's always vigilant with Daniel and expects so much from anyone who's with him. It's hard to accept that we have such little control — that there are no guarantees to keep him safe.

With Alyssa back in town, Joel and I steal some time to get away overnight to the cottage. As we drive up north, we talk almost non-stop, mostly about the kids. Jonathan seems livelier now that his sister is home. We're grateful, too, that even though she must focus on her own need to get better, she is generous with helping her brothers.

Our talk turns to Daniel, who is still our most pressing concern.

We evaluate his progress, trying to predict what his needs will be, and plan how we can best meet them. Joel has a marvellous way of challenging him just enough to guarantee success, and he's able to find the right tone and words to satisfy Daniel when issues arise. Sometimes I wish that there were a manual I could read so I'd know what to do in the moment, too. Like that day when Daniel told me he wanted to have sex with a friend who was coming over to visit that afternoon. Practically choking on my words, certain that the girl in question was just a platonic friend, I searched for a way to dissuade my son.

Whatever I managed to say worked, but Joel's advice to him later that day was more direct, "Daniel, you need to concentrate on getting better. You don't have time for a girlfriend right now."

Getting away is a welcome respite. The weather is pleasantly warm for late April. In spite of pockets of snow that linger in patches beneath the trees, brave tufts of grass are starting to green. There's a hint of spring in the air. At dinner, Joel and I sit outside on the sun porch and watch the clear surface of the lake reflecting the shimmering sunset and the deep shadows of trees. We enter the quiet, allowing the calm of this place to soothe us.

Joel absent-mindedly strokes his beard that is just starting to grey at the tip of his chin. Leaning closer to him, I swirl my fingers along his arm. We need each other so much. I couldn't imagine getting through this without him.

May 15, 1994
Dear Family and Friends,

Daniel continues to stay at Hugh MacMillan Rehabilitation Centre during the week and comes home on weekends. In the past six weeks, many changes have occurred. Several weeks ago, Daniel's vocal cords started to function, giving him a voice. At first he sounded very robotic, like an old computer voice synthesizer. Although his voice is still not normal, we are all so excited with this milestone event. The use of a voice has given Daniel greater control of his environment. It has opened up the doors of communication with staff and peers and has enabled him to express his thoughts and wishes with greater understanding from his listeners.

When he first used his voice in the resource room, his teacher suggested that he call his father at the office. Daniel left a brief message on Joel's voice mail and Joel was so delighted that he kept replaying it all afternoon. As Daniel has gained breath control and some inflection, his voice quality is improving somewhat. He has even begun to sing, but unfortunately no improvement in tone quality is noted compared to his pre-injury ability. It must be that Garmaise gene that was inherited from his grandfather.

Physically, Daniel shows significant improvement. Although he still is confined to a wheelchair, he is learning how to walk with a specialized cane — a quad cane that has a platform and four legs. Last Friday night, I was surprised when I answered the doorbell and found my husband and son standing at the door. Daniel had abandoned his wheelchair and "walked" into the house (closely supervised by Joel). My son sat down in a regular chair in the dining room and was delighted with himself. This weekend, he walked down the stairs to the basement holding onto the railing with his left hand. He was able to stand by himself and maintain his balance while throwing a small basketball. Then he climbed onto an exercise bike and pedalled for ten minutes. Later in the day, he walked back upstairs with his quad cane.

While he has learned to negotiate the hallways of Hugh Mac in his wheelchair and is able to travel independently on the elevator to attend his therapies, he still requires supervision for all day-to-day activities. The impulsivity and impaired judgement that usually follow a head injury are frightening safety issues.

Daniel is so motivated in all his therapies and activities and is getting such positive feedback. We can't believe how hard he's working. He expends so much energy, but still fatigues easily and requires two naps a day. He doesn't always recognize when he's getting tired, but can be seen to fade like a flickering light bulb. Usually Daniel maintains a really upbeat mood. However, at times he expresses feelings of sadness or anger. The music therapy program is a wonderful medium for him as he composes lyrics to express his feelings. He uses the keyboard, drums, and his harmonica.

At a recent conference I attended called "Full Spectrum of Head

Injury," one speaker summed up our feelings, "Hope and fear, fear and hope." We're seeing so much progress and we're grateful and encouraged, but our son still has a long, long way to go. We're still trying to live one day at a time.

Love,

Lainie

CHAPTER THIRTY-TWO

It's a beautiful day, unseasonably warm for May. After the rainy weather we've been having, it's too nice to spend indoors.

"How about some ice cream?" I ask Daniel. "We can drive to the plaza."

Daniel readily agrees. He seldom refuses the offer of food.

We sit outside the Baskin Robbins store, relaxing in the sun like turtles on a rock. As I lick my cone, my mouth fills with the crunch of almonds embedded in smooth pistachio. I'm almost finished; Daniel is much slower. His tongue extends deliberately to lick the ice cream, but he's lost the knack of twirling his cone around to catch the drips. Between my bench and his wheelchair, a small black dog laps up the spills from the ground.

Around us there's a hubbub of activity. People have shed their warm bulky clothing and have sprouted wheels instead — bikers, roller-bladers, parents pushing strollers. Everyone swiftly gliding by. Two girls, in tight T-shirts and even tighter jeans, whisper to one another as they walk past us quickly without any sign of recognition.

"I know them," Daniel says. He waves his cone in their direction and dribbles a splotch of ice cream onto his shirt.

"Maybe they didn't see you," I reply, dabbing at the mess with a napkin. "Who are they?"

"From school. Let's say hello."

I look up and see them zip around the corner. "Too late. They're gone." I pause and reflect a moment about their speed. Shrugging my shoulders, I continue, "Why don't you finish up? And while you're at it, I'll just scoot over to the bakery for some bread."

Dashing out of the store with my purchase, I notice the tight-jeaned girls again. They're peeking around the corner, paying no attention to the displays of photographs and picture frames in the camera shop window.

"He's still there," one says, checking to see if the coast is clear. The other leans back against the window and groans.

What are they afraid of? I want to say something to them, tell them what it would mean to him for them to be friendly, even for just a moment. Words fail me. I'm hurt, discouraged, and angry. I whip past the girls, ignoring them, clutching my bag of bread.

When I get back, Daniel suggests heading in the direction I've just come from. I hustle him towards the car instead. The bright sunshine has suddenly lost its glitter for me.

CHAPTER THIRTY-THREE

On Thursday, June 9, the day before her back surgery, my mother phones. "I think I'll postpone the operation. I'm worried about Dad. He hasn't been well."

"Mom, you've been waiting for months for this surgery, living in constant pain. You have to have it now."

"But what if he dies and I'm not with him?"

"Don't worry. I'll take care of him for you. I promise he won't die while you're in the hospital."

Such foolish words. But they have the desired effect of calming her. The next day I'm more worried about her than him as she's wheeled away on a gurney. She looks so old and frail. Her hand, freckled with brown spots, pats mine reassuringly.

"Don't worry. I'll be fine," she tells me.

I try not to think of what can go wrong. If you don't put words to your fears, maybe they'll remain hidden, unrealized. But, the spectres accompany me to the waiting room. They stare back at me from the ceiling tiles, from the polished floor, play hide-and-seek behind the large philodendron plant in the brass container in the corner of the room. I thought I'd get used to it, this waiting. I've had so much practice.

My brother, Yaron, comes dashing in.

"Am I late? Hear anything yet?"

"No, the doctor said the procedure would take over an hour."

"Then let's go to the coffee shop," he says. "I could use something to eat."

Munching on a muffin, he tells me about the morning meeting he's just come from and the problems he's having hiring a competent assistant. I sip my tea slowly while the phantoms fade, held at bay by the steady flow of his words.

Sunday, two days post-surgery, my mom is recuperating. Her feisty nature is returning too. She'll no longer use a bedpan and insists on getting up to go to the washroom. I'm grateful that at least she's willing to allow the nurses to help. There's already talk of transferring her to a rehabilitation centre for physiotherapy treatment. We fill out forms, listing three options closest to her home. It's unlikely she'll get her favourite choice. She'll have to take whatever placement first becomes available.

When I visit my father that afternoon, I'm surprised to find him lying under the covers of his bed, his pale blue pyjama top a signal that something's amiss. Where's his usual outfit? The bright sweatshirts or sweaters I've grown accustomed to? Today his face is gaunt, his cheeks sunken. His ruddy complexion has faded, making him look like a whitish apparition.

"Hi, Dad. It's Lainie," I say. "Do you want to get up?"

Slowly he turns his head in my direction, blinks his eyes, and silently shakes his head. I plop down in the chair beside him and watch his gaze move back to the ceiling. His left hand lies limply on top of the blanket, the skin as translucent as a sheet of white tissue paper. I tuck his hand under the covers. It feels so cold.

Please don't die now, I think to myself. I promised Mom you wouldn't die while she was in the hospital. Those silly words resound in my ears.

I sit silently as time passes. Five minutes? Ten? It feels like an eternity before I stand and tenderly stroke my father's face goodbye.

At the payphone in the lobby, I rustle in my wallet for a quarter to call my brother.

"What should we tell Mom?" I ask. "She knows I was planning to visit Dad today and she has a right to know how he is."

Yaron says he'll tell her in person; he and Sue will be seeing her later. Then we face a more difficult decision — should we ask Amichai to come back from Israel?

"Let's wait," Yaron suggests. "See what happens."

Days pass with no improvement in my father's condition. He's completely bedridden and is no longer taking any food. The doctor has told us that all she can do is to keep him hydrated and medicated for pain.

We wait.

On Wednesday, my mother transfers from the hospital to St. Bernard's, a Catholic rehabilitation facility. Strange to find a rehab centre that's not easily accessible; the front door is flanked by a flight of stairs. An attendant pulls my mother's wheelchair backwards up the steeply sloped receiving ramp. We wait on the landing for the buzzer to be answered by a nun who leads us to the reception area. The foyer is spotless, the floor and woodwork polished as if by a legion of invisible elves. In front of the window, two huge dieffenbachia plants flourish, stretching their broad gleaming leaves upward in supplication. Soon another nun leads us to an elevator that creaks its way to the second floor. I follow her into my mother's assigned room. The room, shared with another patient, is tiny, the two beds so close it's hard to manoeuvre her wheelchair. My mother is upset to find a cross hanging over her bed.

"This isn't where I wanted to be," she whimpers.

"I know," I whisper back. "I'll see what I can do."

The head nurse listens sympathetically. Tomorrow she'll move my mother into a private room, one where we can detach the cross or cover it up without offending anyone.

When I go to visit my father Thursday evening, I can hear the unevenness of his breath before I enter his room. It sounds so laboured, a whistling catch in his throat that can't be cleared and then silence, before he gurgles once more. I want the familiar rhythm like the steady chugging of a train that pushes hard, even up a steep hill.

I can't bear to walk in.

With tears streaming down my face, I lean against the doorway and whisper, "Goodbye, Dad. I love you."

It's my last visit.

My mother is not looking forward to spending the weekend at the rehab centre. There's no therapy available, yet she knows she can't go home. She's champing at the bit by the time I visit late Saturday morning.

"Let's go outside," I suggest.

I wheel her down the gently sloping ramp, the one we hadn't noticed before, at the far end of the front lobby. The grounds at the back of the centre are extensive and the gardens look lovingly cared for. Borders of glistening periwinkle, pinks, and purple-stalked ajuga embrace the winding paved pathways. Interspersed in the perennial beds are sprays of annuals adding a splash of colour, while bowers of shade trees offer an invitation to rest on wrought-iron benches. The garden is calming. A good place to wait.

We're waiting for the anticipated yet dreaded phone call with news of my father. It's time.

Time also for Amichai to come. When he arrives on Monday afternoon, Yaron drives him directly from the airport to visit Mom. Then my brothers go together to visit Dad. A few hours after that visit, a nurse calls to tell me my father has died. I don't know whether I believe in fate, but I wonder if Dad was waiting for Amichai to arrive so we could all be together to face his departure. Maybe he needed to hear his son's voice giving him permission to leave us. Like a good soldier, he was just waiting for his marching orders to come through.

It's shortly before 10:00 p.m. when my brothers, Sue, and I turn up at St. Bernard's Rehab Centre. Visiting hours ended at 8:30 p.m. and the place is closed tighter than a drum. We ring the bell and wait on the doorstep for the nun on duty to let us in. The hallway rings hollowly, echoing our footsteps as we walk down the corridor to the nursing station on the second floor. When we explain our purpose, the nurse, worried about my mother's reaction, offers to come with us and softly knocks on the door. My mother is sitting in a chair reading.

"The time has come, Mom," Amichai says, taking hold of her hand and leading her to the bed where they both sit down. We gather round, encircling them. Unobtrusively, the nurse disappears, closing the door behind her.

As we begin to answer her questions, my mother's shoulders relax. The tenseness, the holding, the waiting for the worst to happen is gone now — released. Her husband is finally at peace.

"It's okay," she says, patting my hand, silently forgiving me for my unfulfilled promise. "A blessing really. I was spared the worst." Her touch feels firmer now. "When I said goodbye to him ten days ago, he was still all right. I can hold onto that memory instead of the ghostly image that you must have." She inhales deeply and lies back against the pillows. "How can I make any arrangements from here?"

"You don't have to do a thing," Yaron says.

"All you have to do is rest and concentrate on getting yourself better." Amichai rises to leave. "I'll see you in the morning."

Our family gathers around us for the funeral. My father's brother David, the only surviving sibling of ten, has come from Chicago, and three of my mother's four sisters and their husbands are here from New York, Rhode Island, and Florida.

I feel sorry for Jonathan. He has never been to a funeral before and doesn't know what to expect. When Joel's father died suddenly last summer, Jonathan was away on a six-day canoe trip in Algonquin Park and unreachable by phone, so he didn't join us until several days later. Today Jonathan looks handsome in his new suit, the one we bought for his junior high school graduation scheduled tonight. He won't be going.

"I know it's not fair," I say.

Jonathan nods in agreement, poker-faced.

The funeral director pins black ribbons on the immediate family members and makes a snip in each to indicate grief. We stand for the K'reeah ceremony, the rending of the ribbon, which teaches us to meet all sorrow standing upright. My mother, briefly erect beside her wheelchair, appears stalwart. She's grateful that the rabbi from our former synagogue in Montreal will be in charge today. He knows us well, and feels like a family member, too. From officiating at our bar and bat mitzvahs, to weddings, and now to my father's funeral, Rabbi Leffell has shared a full circle of life with us.

When the service is about to begin, Yaron wheels my mother into the funeral hall. Amichai and I take our places near her, and my uncle and the rest of the family follow. Glancing around, I notice the familiar faces of friends and colleagues, as people continue to settle into their seats. The room is nearly full and a hush descends like the quiet in a symphony hall as the conductor approaches the podium. Daniel has just entered the room.

He's not in a wheelchair today; he's walking, using a cane, and guided by his father.

Whispers and gasps of amazement fill the hall. In the midst of our sadness, we have something to celebrate.

That evening at my home, another unexpected celebration. My friend Gerri, our school trustee, drops by, inviting us all out to the front porch where she formally presents Jonathan with his junior high school certificate. Still dressed in his suit, my youngest son accepts the scrolled document from her. Smiling, he shakes her hand. I take a photo for our family album, certain my father would approve.

The *shiva* is being held at my home. We've curtailed the hours for this week of mourning since my mother still needs therapy, and isn't able to sit for any extended period of time. We're trying to accommodate Daniel's needs, too. We consider him so vulnerable. Joel is afraid of turning him into a spectacle, yet I believe it's important for him to be here with us. We've talked of having him sleep at home this week with Joel driving him back to Hugh Mac each morning. Meanwhile, my brothers and I have decided to attend morning services at the synagogue; in the evenings we'll hold them at the house with friends and family members joining in.

Our friends are generous with their support, providing evening meals for us. With my extended family at the table, each dinner feels somewhat like a festive meal despite the underlying note of sorrow. My father would have loved to join in. He always used get-togethers as an opportunity to retell the tales that we had heard so many times before.

One evening during the *shiva,* Alyssa introduces me to a young man named Adam, who's come to pay his respects. His features seem nondescript, a pleasant face topped with light brown curls, not someone I expect to remember. There have been many strangers showing kindness this week.

"I just met Alyssa a few weeks ago and she told me about her brother. I've had a brain injury too," he says. "Two years ago. Now I'm back at university."

I look at him more closely. He shows no physical handicaps and his cognition is obviously good. He's definitely one of the lucky ones.

"Would it be okay if I talk with Daniel?" Adam asks. "I'd like to give him some encouragement."

"Yes, I'd like that," I say.

When Adam leaves, I'm startled to see him get into a car and drive away. It seems too farfetched to imagine my son driving again, yet if I had a crystal ball and could look two years ahead, I would see Daniel behind the wheel of a car once more.

June 27, 1994
Dear Family and Friends,

Daniel's progress has been incredible of late. Each weekend when he comes home, we notice new things that he can do in all realms: physical, cognitive, and emotional. He still uses his wheelchair in the rehab centre to get to and from his therapies, but at home on weekends he walks using a cane. This weekend he set himself the goal of walking to the corner of our street, a distance of 300 metres. He was so proud to reach the stop sign — a new milestone.

For months, we have learned to celebrate any small changes that occurred. Now we're watching him become much more aware of his abilities and limitations. During a recent meeting with the psychologist at Hugh Mac, Daniel started to express his anger at the driver of the car and his sadness at the part of himself that has been lost. The therapists are so pleased with this breakthrough. It's important for him to begin the grieving process before he can move on, but it's so painful for us to see. We've had a long time to cry and grieve. Now it's his turn.

He's concerned about his future and asks about school and work. What will I be able to do? How long will this take?

We have to help him separate his negative feelings from the positive ones that he applies to his rehabilitation. No one can believe how motivated and determined he is!

With new abilities come new challenges. He is seeking to regain as much independence as he can, but safety is still the prime consideration. He has learned to go to the washroom independently, but the nursing staff still provide supervision while attempting to respect his privacy. At a recent swallow clinic, the decision was made to allow him unsupervised eating. This means that he can now eat in the kid's cafeteria at Hugh Mac rather than in the solarium under the supervision of the nursing staff. He's never quite understood the concern of the nurses: for weeks now, he's been surreptitiously eating snacks brought by his friends with no ill effects. He even tried to negotiate with one of the doctors, and offered to give up the permission to chew gum in exchange for drinking thin liquids. However, the latter requires another videofluoroscopy to ensure that no silent aspiration of liquids is occurring. This test will probably take place sometime in July. Meanwhile, he continues with thickened fluids.

Our weekends remain focussed on extending our son's rehab. We do electrical stimulation on his right leg and exercises for his leg and right arm. He practises writing with his left hand, and we engage him in functional tasks such as meal preparation and loading the dishwasher in addition to cognitive activities like game playing and planning his own leisure time. He's made huge gains, but has a long way to go on the path to independent living.

Recently, our family spent a weekend at the cottage with two of Daniel's friends. It was exciting to take him out in the boat and see how much he recalled. He knew his way around the lake and pointed out landmarks, like our previous cottage and those of several neighbours. He knew how to get to the various marinas and gave directions on how to navigate correctly through the buoy system. As the weather was very warm, he even got to go swimming with a life jacket on. He had such a good time that he was reluctant to come out of the lake.

Last week, I discussed with Daniel his grandfather's imminent death to find out whether he wanted to be involved in the mourning process. I explained about the funeral, the visit to the cemetery, and the *shiva*. I warned him that the mourners might be in tears and it could be upsetting for him. He replied, "I'll be there to give you a hug." During this past week he's been talking to the visitors who have come to pay their respects and relating well to them. We're so pleased with his progress and when we see the sparkle that has returned to his eyes, we truly believe that more is to come.

Love,

Laini

CHAPTER THIRTY-FOUR

The radio is turned off and my husband and I talk sparingly as we drive from our cottage to Haliburton. It's a familiar route — part highway, part winding country road — to the camp where Daniel used to be a counsellor. Sometimes I treasure silence — the quiet hush when my family is asleep and I can tiptoe outside into a summer night where sparkling stars wrap around me like a beaded shawl. I love the tranquillity of a cold winter's day with just the crackle of burning logs in the fireplace and a rustling newspaper to disturb the calm. Smiling, I think of years of companionable silences that Joel and I have shared while walking along a beach, through the woods, or just resting on the couch after a long day's work. This July day, however, our wordlessness is a sign of our preoccupation.

Alyssa called us when she picked Daniel up from the rehab

centre. They're going to meet us at the hotel, and tomorrow we'll see Jonathan at camp. Despite her encouragement, Daniel refused to take his wheelchair. Nothing she said could get him to change his mind. He wouldn't even let her pack it in the trunk, just in case. He didn't anticipate any "just in case." It didn't really surprise me, but left me wondering what the weekend will bring.

When the cellphone rings again, I'm anticipating a further problem. Instead I'm delighted to hear Jonathan's voice.

"Hi, Mom. Come and get me."

"What? Where are you?"

"At camp. Just came back from a five-day canoe trip. The director said I could come to the hotel and have dinner with you guys. So pick me up right now, okay? That way I won't have to wait in line for the camp showers."

Twenty minutes later, Jonathan is bubbling and gurgling as excitedly as a spring brook. With his words, he paints pictures of a mist rising at dawn from the lake to reveal a huge moose feeding placidly near the shoreline. I can practically feel the cold spray of the waterfall he paddled near and the heat of the campfire he huddled beside each dusk, trying to avoid mosquito attacks. He spins more and more tales, as wound up as a top. We listen eagerly. When we check into the hotel, he reluctantly quiets down.

Our room is darkened, the curtains drawn, and Daniel is alone in the room, asleep. Jonathan dashes for the shower and we stroll over to the coffee shop, looking for Alyssa. We wait for her to finish her snack, then saunter back to the room together. She's walking again, her rental wheelchair returned, but she tells us her joints feel stiff from the long drive.

"Let's all go swimming," she says.

A blaring TV greets our return, loud enough to drown out Niagara Falls. Daniel is awake.

It's only a short distance from the terrace complex to the main hotel building, yet we drive there, trying to conserve Daniel's energy. Joel leads the boys to the change room and Alyssa goes on ahead, too. Walking through the lobby, I spot Allison, a friend of Daniel's. She rushes over to me, gushing with news of all the camp counsellors who've arranged their day off at this hotel so they could see their friend. They've just started to arrive. In carloads of three and four they emerge, coming straight to the pool where Daniel is seated under an umbrella. There are more than a dozen of them. I'm concerned that Daniel will be overwhelmed, but Allison acts as mistress of ceremonies, quietly cueing him to names as different people approach him. Squealing girls slather him with kisses; guys pump his left arm. Daniel just sits there, nodding and grinning with pleasure.

He doesn't notice when the sky darkens to an uneasy grey. Soon droplets of rain begin to splatter, ping, ping, bouncing off the ledge of the pool. Alyssa, Jonathan, and Joel, the only ones in the water, scurry out to get changed. The rest of us move into the lounge where Daniel continues to hold court. Sitting out of the way in a corner of the room, I listen as snippets of conversation buzz around me like bees in a field of flowers: Phil is talking to Daniel, Alyssa is back and chatting with Rachel. Jonathan plays pool with some fellow I don't know. Joel joins me.

The counsellors begin to clear out, setting off to their rooms to rest, shower, or grab a bite to eat. We go to the hotel's café for dinner and get a table for five.

From the middle of the room come peals of laughter from a group of guys. Their mirth and delight seem contagious, but instead I'm saddened, wishing that Daniel were still part of the group. He would have been on ski staff again this summer and was hoping to take over as head of water-skiing in a few years' time. The food catches in my throat as I try to swallow the would-have-beens and should-have-beens.

Towards the end of our dinner, we see Phil and Rachel waiting for a table. When they're seated, Jonathan gets up to join them, and we suggest that Daniel take his coffee over to sit with them, too. We hear talk of the counsellors going to The Beak, a local bar where the younger ones sneak in with their fake I.D. Alyssa decides to join them, but Daniel can't. He's already fading and can't even hang out in the lounge with his friends after dinner.

Joel drives us back to the room, where I supervise Daniel's preparations for bed. Jonathan must return to camp now. When my husband returns, he finds me sitting in the silent room, staring out at the dark through the open chink in the curtain. Daniel's asleep, and it's not yet 9:00 p.m.

Shortly after breakfast on Saturday, Phil and Rachel meet in our room. They want to be with Daniel to see his reaction when he visits camp. We divide our group into two cars, and drive through Haliburton, a small town with a long main street and not much else. Phil acts as a tour guide, pointing out landmarks that would be meaningful to his friend. Daniel slowly turns his head from side to side looking at the ice cream shop, laundromat, supermarket, and the tour highlight — McKeck's, the local restaurant with greasy home fries and the best wings around. At the town's main set of traffic lights, we turn right. Soon we're driving up the winding dirt road to camp, passing pretty lakeside cottages and an old quarry site where piles of rust-coloured earth are all that remain of former industry.

Today's visit is different from previous ones. This time, we're allowed to drive directly into camp. On visitor's day, we always joined a long procession of cars filled with parents, siblings, and barking dogs. Counsellors in green T-shirts emblazoned with STAFF in thick white lettering directed us to park far down the roadway if we weren't early enough to get one of the coveted spots on the empty softball field. Behind the stone gates the older campers crowded, pretending they didn't care when their families showed up, yet their squeals of delight belied their nonchalant manner. I remember the time that Daniel sat perched on top of the stone gateway itself. Was he fourteen or fifteen then? It seems so long ago.

Joel stops the car as close as he can to cabin B9 and I hop out to open the door for Daniel. Slowly he slides his left hand under his right knee to lift up his foot. With deliberation, he swings first one foot and then the other onto the ground. Then, leaning on his cane, he tries to stand. I reach out my arm to steady my son as he plants his legs wide apart, balancing precariously on the uneven terrain. He reminds me a little of the four-foot high inflatable clown my brothers and I played with as kids. Its fat grin and laughing eyes never wavered. No matter how hard we punched it, it kept popping back up for more.

"Guys, come on over," someone calls. "Look who's here. It's Daniel!"

A sea of friendly faces immediately surrounds him.

"Hey, man, what's up?"

"Whatcha been doing with yourself?"

"Remember me? I was in the next cabin, B8."

Daniel looks around bewildered, mute. Joel presses close to his side. In the wake of the silence, some of the staff become flustered, shifting awkwardly from one leg to the other.

Someone says, "Well, it's been good to see you."

And Daniel says, "Good to see you, too."

The tension is broken when two female counsellors come running towards us. They throw their arms around him, and he kisses each on a cheek.

"Wow, Dan, you look great," one says.

"Have you been in your old cabin yet?" the second asks. "No? Well, let's go then."

We follow her into the counsellors' cubicle. A thin curtain over a narrow doorway separates this area from the campers' portion of the cabin. It feels cramped in this small rectangle with its two sets of bunk beds. Three of the beds are unmade and the fourth one looks out of place with its neat covering. Sporting equipment floats suspended from the rafters, clothing rests in wobbly piles on open wooden shelves, and over it all hangs the musty smell of sweaty socks and damp towels drooping from nails. In one corner near the window, a large boom box has been hooked up with extra speakers to drown the place in music. Mercifully, it's quiet now.

Daniel smiles as he points to the top bunk on the right hand side of the room near the doorway.

"I slept here," he tells us, delighting in the revival of memory.

"Yeah, right, when you weren't hiding out in Bunk 10 to skip breakfast and catch some extra sleep," Phil says.

"Don't deny it, man. You were the best at sneaking away to catch twenty winks," says another counsellor.

My son's puzzled expression suggests that not all camp memories are going to be retrieved.

Our next stop is the camp office, where the director and his wife greet Daniel warmly.

"Let's go outside to talk," Cecily says, inviting him to fill them in about his progress.

We sit on the wooden porch overlooking the lake and the waterfront. Blue-green water blends into blue sky; the green spatters along the shoreline in emerald trees and jade bushes. From the docks below us drift the sounds of splashing and children's laughter.

Just then, Steve, the co-head of water-skiing, bounds up the stairs and offers his friend a high five. "I was just coming to ask if we could take you out in the ski boat." He turns to the camp director. "Would that be all right? Yes? Great! Let's move it then. Richie is waiting for us at the dock."

I stand watching on the porch. Daniel's cane scrapes against stones as he tries to secure purchase on the uneven surface. The rasping sound sends shivers up my arms, as grating as a fingernail scraped on a classroom blackboard. When the cane prongs slip again,

Daniel leans heavily on his father's arm. They look like a set of Siamese twins joined that way, and together they plod to the dock. But the performance hasn't ended yet. There's still the production of getting Daniel into the boat — helping him into a kneeling position, then lowering his buttocks until he's seated and his legs are dangling over the side of the dock. The gap between his feet and the floorboard must be negotiated so Joel and Steve hold him steady, carefully guiding him into the boat. With Daniel settled, Steve waves to Jonathan to hop in.

Richie revs the engine and the boat takes off with a roar. It cuts through the water with barely a wake, its hull designed to skim the surface like a dragonfly skittering across the rippling lake. Standing on the pier with his arms crossed, Joel stares out at the receding boat. From my perch, I watch, too. Alyssa, Rachel, and Phil cluster nearby. Brushing my eyes with the back of my hand, I listen to Phil's running commentary.

"They're heading over to the slalom course now. Can you see those orange balls in the distance? Towards the right. Did you know that last summer Daniel set the record for the fastest speed through the course? Thirty-six miles an hour! Can you believe it? No one's beaten it yet this year. Of course, no one else has his special ski — his Kidder Red Line. He loved that ski. Treated it like a baby. Thought it better than any O'Brien or Connelly, and not just any Kidder would do. It had to be the Red Line."

My eyes follow Phil's outstretched arm to the bouncing orange balls. The only thing missing right now is the skier.

July 25, 1994

Dear Phil and Rachel,

This weekend was so special for Daniel and I wanted to write to thank you. Having so many of the Timberlane Staff at the hotel on Friday was such an exciting experience for him. I felt that he was practically holding court with so many friends surrounding him in the lounge. And I know that he really enjoyed sitting with you in the restaurant and spending the day with you on Saturday.

Saturday was a very exciting day for Dan. He was so pleased to recognize camp and to find things were familiar to him. Although the terrain was rough going, he enjoyed sitting on the porch at the main beach and especially going for that boat ride with Steve and Richie. Jonathan said that Daniel had a grin from ear to ear, and he keeps talking about how they drove through the slalom course at his speed: 36 m.p.h. He's absolutely determined to ski again, and I believe that he will do it. On Sunday morning for the first time, all the fingers of his right hand were moving. Alyssa feels that this is more than a mere coincidence. If he wants to ski his right hand will have to work.

I found Saturday an emotionally draining experience. Daniel should be in camp surrounded by his friends and I was so sad that he's not there. I also found it hard to talk to his friends about their plans for university in the fall knowing that Daniel would have gone, too. When we watched him through those months in Sunnybrook, we would not have anticipated even this. I'm thankful that he could visit camp, but once he's made it this far, we all want so much more for him. More importantly, he wants it for himself. We just have to keep hoping and believing that it will happen.

Daniel is going to be at the cottage with us during the first week in August. If you have a day off during that time and want to spend it with us, we'd be delighted to have you. Our guest cabin is like a villa — beds for five but lots of floor space, and the price is right. We've mentioned this to Allison, Larry, Adam, Steve, and Richie. Other friends would also be more than welcome, of course. I realize that transportation and distance is a drawback, one and a half hours of driving in each direction, but do let us know if you plan to come. You have the cottage number.

If we don't see you, continue to have a great summer and keep an eye on Jonathan for us.

Fondly,
Lainie Cohen

August 8, 1994
Dear Family and Friends,

We've just spent a week vacationing at the cottage with Dan. Alyssa joined us on weekends; Jonathan is still at camp. The staff at Hugh Mac may have hoped that we would just relax, but they should have realized by now how intense and driven Joel and I are when it comes to Daniel's rehabilitation. In addition to the normal daily routines of muscle stimulation for his ankle, leg exercises, right arm exercises, and mouth exercises to help with enunciation, we came equipped for cognitive and academic rehabilitation.

Hugh Mac's academic resource program shuts down in August so we decided to replicate it. I borrowed some workbooks from the teacher who will be tutoring Daniel this month and bought some new games and computer programs. One of Daniel's goals is to return to school to finish his one remaining high school credit, so he is highly motivated to engage in reading and math activities to regain his skills. Cognitive deficits in attention and memory have had a significant impact on these skills. The workbooks constituted the "work" aspect of our program, but the games just seemed like fun.

Daniel has no difficulty learning or relearning how to play games: checkers, Othello, gin, cribbage, euchre, Monopoly, Telepaths, Scruples — the list goes on and on. The cottage is a natural environment for games where age limits don't matter. One day, a neighbour — visiting with her five-year-old daughter — brought over a Chinese checkers game. Daniel had a great time playing with the little girl, who insisted on sitting beside him when they stayed for dinner. Aha, a new female conquest! He even prepared her chocolate milk.

While on the topic of liquids, Daniel's latest videofluoroscopy in July indicated that he could drink non-thickened fluids. I'm certain that the profits of Coke have risen significantly since. It's great to be able to take Daniel into a restaurant where he can order anything he wants.

We tried to include some special activities in our holiday. We took Daniel out to dinner and to a play in Gravenhurst, to a movie in Bracebridge, and to Bala for a frozen yogurt and mini-golf. I think one of Daniel's highlights was just going with Robert, Alyssa, and her friend Michelle to the nearest grocery store in Torrance to pick out a video. What a normal thing to do — four young adults and no parents at all.

So many highlights mark this week of holiday. Daniel was able to swim on his back without any lifejacket or aid all the way from our dock to our neighbour's and back (with Joel alongside, of course). He and Joel walked up our long driveway to a cottage that is three houses down the road. The best was the morning when Joel and I left him alone for the first time since his injury. As parents we're trying to ensure his safety while having to learn to let go. Joel had gone to play golf and I went to take my daily hour-long walk. Our son was delighted to be unsupervised while he went through his morning routines of washing, shaving, dressing, and walking downstairs for breakfast. What a step towards independence! There will be many more to follow.

We have learned to celebrate every step of progress with wonder and excitement. We desperately try to stay focussed on the day-to-day events and not project too far ahead. What an impossible task — especially as Daniel's view of his progress is so global. Being able to open the fridge with his right hand while holding a container of orange juice in his left hand after walking without a cane for the few steps from counter to fridge is merely a minor accomplishment in his eyes.

As we watch him rebuild step by step to what he will be, his goal is perfect recovery to what he was.

"When will my right hand work properly? How long will I need this leg brace? When will I go back to school? When I water-ski, will I be able to cut the wake the way I used to?"

We try to explain that no one knows these answers, not even the doctors or therapists. He'll just have to keep working hard, and we'll be there to help him.

Love,

Lainie

Part Three

CHAPTER THIRTY-FIVE

I carry my bowl of bran flakes and the container of milk onto the sun porch of the cottage, set it down on the table, and gaze at the early-morning lake. A light breeze ripples the surface. Near the shoreline, my turquoise canoe straddles two logs that keep it suspended above the ground. I ignore the canoe's silent beckoning. I haven't used it once all summer, and now it's almost Labour Day, my last chance. But there's no time. No time for many of the things I'd like to do — at least that's how it feels. As I eat, my mind races with all the chores still left for this weekend: remove the perishables from the fridge, make sure that all the food in the pantry is in airtight containers to keep out the mice, and remember to pack the woollen blankets in thick plastic bags. It's always like this at the end of the summer: a lot of hustle and bustle.

During the day, when the sky is whitewashed with streaks of thin cloud, we watch as motorboats race by with skiers, and jet skis zoom non-stop past our dock. Other cottagers seem determined to cram as much fun as possible into these waning days of vacation. The cooler water temperature doesn't deter Daniel, but the rest of us don't want to linger in the lake. We won't be back much after this weekend. We plan to leave tomorrow right after breakfast. Joel delays the task of putting away deck chairs and life jackets until the sun starts to fade. At dusk, the trees look pasted on the horizon like stage scenery — dark cardboard cutouts that will soon vanish from view.

This summer has had a persistent drone to it. Joel and I are focussed on Daniel's rehabilitation, on Daniel's needs. It's how we define our days. When other family members are around, I feel like a juggler trying to keep all the balls in the air. Am I the only one who struggles with balance?

Jonathan seems to be more himself, the way he used to be before Daniel's injury — bouncy and excited by his experience at summer camp. It was good for Jonathan to get a break from his brother for a while, and from all our other problems, too. When Jonathan came home, he told us he made some new friends at camp, friends who will be starting high school with him. I hope he does well in grade ten. A new school, a fresh slate, a time for new possibilities.

Alyssa is bouncing back too. All those physiotherapy sessions have helped. Although she didn't get to work this summer as planned, she's feeling much better now and is ready to return to university for her senior year to finish off her business degree. She and her friend Marni are eager to meet their new roommate, an exchange student from Finland who'll be with them for the fall semester.

Even my mother is doing better. She's spent a lot of weekends up north with us this summer. At first, she was reluctant to come, worried that she'd be too much of a burden on me as she needed help to get in and out of the shower and to walk down to the dock. But she's recuperated well from her back surgery last June, and has regained her independence. Daniel enjoys having his grandmother around because she's always willing to drop what she's doing whenever he approaches with a deck of cards. Yet, sometimes when she's with him, I can see her smile flicker and her eyes shadow with fading dreams.

I know my mother misses Dad, but she doesn't talk about him much. She's been living alone as a quasi-widow for several years already and has a strong network of friends. She'll keep busy. Her spirited nature guarantees it.

I'm reluctant to go home. As the first day of school draws near, I usually feel a sense of excitement. I can remember looking forward each September to the scent of freshly waxed hallways, the brightness of posters lining bulletin boards, the gleam of clean chalkboards, and freshly scrubbed faces. September always brings a heightened sensation of opportunity.

This year is different. I feel out of sync with my part-time work schedule, and it's hard to get my mind tuned into work. It's really the uncertainty that bothers me. I'm worried that I may have to give up my job completely to become Daniel's attendant/chauffeur when he's discharged from the rehab centre. We've talked of hiring someone to do these tasks, but I remember how difficult it was to find someone to take care of him for just a few hours on a weekend when we wanted a break. I don't feel very confident about finding someone we can trust.

My mood has been down since last Monday, the anniversary date of Daniel's injury. At the rehab centre, we see other teenagers whose recuperation speeds along at a much faster pace than his. Joel attempted to cheer me up by having us speak to the neurosurgeon who operated on our son. Unfortunately, I was on the line with another call when he tried to patch me into the conference call, so I missed her encouraging remarks. Joel phoned me immediately afterwards and excitedly repeated everything for me.

"Of course, I remember Daniel," she had said. "When I left to take up my new position in the United States, all he could do was pick out jellybeans from a jar. I'm impressed by his progress now. He's gone further in one year than I could have predicted. And I want to remind you that cognitive development is the last to come, especially abstract reasoning skills. Rest assured, there'll be further progress."

I try to hold onto these words as if by repeating them, they'll somehow come true. The power of positive thinking. I add books on this theme to my reading list, hoping to change my mood. In the past, it was easy to appreciate the good things my life contained — there was such an abundance of blessings. Now, with Daniel's trauma, it sometimes feels that the life we're leading is as wobbly as a house of cards, like the ones my brothers and I used to construct in the middle of our living room on rainy afternoons. We'd add each card, balancing it, carefully weighting it against the next, knowing that with one false move the whole structure would collapse. That never deterred us; we'd just pick up the cards and start again. Finally tired of our game, we'd purposefully destroy our creation.

My life is not a deck of cards. I resolve to focus on the positive.

Preparations for the Jewish New Year are time consuming but rewarding. It feels wonderful to be able to be a complete family of five again. In services, we sit near the entrance in a special section reserved for the disabled. I don't care that my husband and sons arrive late and aren't even interested in opening their prayer books. They look the part, all dressed up in their suits and ties, their heads covered with *kippot*, their shoulders with prayer shawls.

Daniel sits beside me. He's overwhelmed by the large crowd of people, and keeps looking around for familiar faces. When he sees a former classmate or a friend from camp, he smiles and waves like a little kid. Suddenly, he hears a voice, a rich tenor with flowing cadences that resound through the speakers.

"I know him," he says, in too loud a whisper.

"Shhh," I say, trying to hush him. "It's the *chazzan* who always sings the prayers."

"See. I still know some things."

Daniel is restless through the rabbi's sermon, which offers too much information for him to process, and is so exhausted by the time we arrive home that he skips our holiday lunch in order to nap. When the serving platters pass by his empty place, I tell myself that at least he's home with us. Last year at this time, he was in a coma in the hospital. We have much to celebrate this New Year.

A day later, we arrange to take Daniel back to Sunnybrook Hospital to visit the occupational therapist who worked with him following his injury. We feel a special connection to Alison. Aside from the neurosurgeon, she was the only staff member who consistently offered us the possibility of hope. At a conference last winter, she made a presentation about the importance of family support in rehabilitation, showing her colleagues a copy of the daily journal we had kept by Daniel's bedside, as well as a video she had made of him. Today, her calm manner explodes into an exuberant hello as she watches him walk into the rehab department using his quad cane.

Daniel looks great. His hair has fully grown in and the scar on his scalp is barely visible. When Alison compliments him, he tells her he's letting his hair grow so he can wear it in a ponytail again.

Alison offers to give him a tour around the department. She shows him the training computer and pulls out some of the activities he used to work on. Daniel is interested in one that looks like a large children's toy. Colourful plastic hoops are looped around the ends of a thick red semi-circle set in a wooden block. My son grasps a blue ring with his right hand and easily lifts it up and over to the other side. I remember when he had trouble using his left hand to do this task. Now, however, he needs his left hand to help him release his grip on the hoop.

When we leave the occupational therapy department, we head to his former ward, where Daniel recognizes two attendants. Proudly, he uses his right hand to shake Abdul's hand, and then chats briefly with Nancy. There aren't any familiar faces at the nursing station. The turnover of nursing staff must be very high. On our way out, I peek into room C157 — his old room. The walls look barren and sterile, the way we left them last January. The brown vinyl chair beneath the window is not at all inviting.

CHAPTER THIRTY-SIX

Victim Impact Statement: another term to add to our vocabulary — this one from the legal setting. A lawyer from the prosecutor's office has been in touch with us and sent us a form to fill out. She's gathering evidence to determine whether to press criminal charges against the driver, Daniel's former friend, John. The charge being considered is "dangerous driving causing bodily harm."

As Joel and I complete the form, I'm struck by the impact Daniel's injury has had not only on him, but on all our family members. Loss of sleep, loss of weight, reduced income, difficulties with focus and attention at school and at work — quantifiable results. But there's so much more that can't be tallied, like counting the grains of sand on a beach. Whenever I hear a siren shrill or see the red lights of an ambulance flash, my stomach clenches. Will another family soon be suffering the same fate as mine?

My mood shifts upward with the approach of Thanksgiving. I'm infused with deep feelings of gratitude as Daniel is being discharged as an in-patient from Hugh MacMillan Centre. He tells me how good it feels to be coming home to live — quite a milestone after thirteen and a half months in institutions. I'm grateful also, that he can keep his bed at the rehab centre to use for naps while he continues there until December as an outpatient.

I've invited our friends, Ellen and Marc and their two sons, to dinner to celebrate. Alyssa is in town with her roommate from Finland, and my mom has joined us too, so we're a large crowd. My mother always fusses when I have lots of guests. I guess she's worried that I'll tire myself, so she's forever jumping out of her seat to help me serve. "The kids can help," I tell her, but she never listens.

The kids are busy, engaged in lively conversation with one another. Even Joel is animated tonight, buoyed by the knowledge that Daniel is home for good.

At the end of the meal, Ellen brings out the dessert she's baked — chocolate mint brownies, Daniel's favourite. He offers to share them with all the dinner guests, then fills his own plate to overflowing. When our guests depart, Joel hides the leftover brownies, concerned that Daniel will show no restraint in eating them. But Daniel won't go to bed until he's found them. Then he chooses a new hiding spot of his own. He promises to ration his intake and even to share them with Jonathan. I'm not sure if he will. I can see the headline now: Sibling rivalry renewed over mint brownies.

I'm on my way to the tailor on Tuesday to drop off a pair of Daniel's jeans with a broken zipper. My attention shifts from the slow-moving traffic to the grocery list I'm composing in my head: milk, bananas, apples, detergent. Is there anything else we need? If this traffic doesn't ease up soon, I won't have time to shop before picking up Daniel at the rehab centre. Today is his first day as an outpatient, and I don't want to be late.

The cellphone interrupts my thoughts.

"Ran a mile," pants Jonathan. "Gym class."

I can barely make out what he's saying; his breath is so shallow and laboured.

"Asthma attack, Mom. My puffer's at home."

"I'll get it and be right there."

While I wait for the red light to change, my heart pounds. Da-dum. Da-dum. Faster and louder than the flicking turn signal. C'mon, c'mon. Let's go.

The red light doesn't budge.

Calm down, I tell myself. Jonathan is okay. If not, his teacher would take him directly to the hospital. But why didn't Jonathan get a lift home? He's closer to the house than I am. Closer to his puffer.

The light changes. I turn left, then pull onto the eastbound ramp of the highway, relieved that the traffic is moving briskly in this direction. Bayview Avenue is just two exits away. I sigh. This isn't a good time for something to go wrong. I was just telling my mother the other day how Jonathan is finally on an even keel. He's been easier to live with since he came home from camp this summer and seems to be doing more for school. When I pass the open doorway of his room, I often see him working at his desk. That's where his puffer is, in the top drawer.

I leave the car running, dash upstairs, and grab it.

It doesn't take me long before I'm in the driveway in front of Jonathan's school. And there he is, sitting on a step, still dressed in his gym shorts. Before I can get out of the car, he bounds towards me. He looks fine now — thank goodness. Swinging his knapsack in one hand, he opens the door and plops into the front seat. His breathing has returned to normal.

"Thanks, Mom," he says warmly. "Can you take me home now?"

"No, sorry. I'm already late for Daniel. We have to pick him up."

Jonathan's smile freezes. For a moment, I'm afraid that he'll retreat into sullen silence. I reach over and pat his leg, surprised by its child-like smoothness. Is it just my imagination or have his legs grown even longer since the summer?

"I'm glad you're okay."

He nods, then starts to chat about his gym class. His voice becomes vibrant as he tells me that he is one of the fastest runners. I remember Joel saying he used to be good at that, too.

In the parking lot of the rehab centre, Jonathan elects to wait in the car. He fiddles with the radio, trying to find a good station, as I hurry off to fetch Daniel. When we return, Jonathan turns off the music and wordlessly gives up the front seat to his older brother, who slowly settles into place. The seatbelt clicks, then Daniel turns around.

"That's my jacket," he says, glaring at Jonathan. "You didn't ask me."

"You weren't supposed to notice. I thought I'd get home before you," Jonathan replies, not bothering to add an apology.

The drive home is a quiet one, fraught with unspoken words.

At home, Jonathan quickly disappears into his room and closes the door, claiming he has homework. Daniel walks into the kitchen with me for a snack. When he prepares a plate of cheese and crackers, I praise his healthy selection. He has to be retaught about nutrition and still monitored while he eats. Because he's less physically active than before his injury, he can't easily burn off those junk food calories that teenagers love to consume. Besides, the nursing staff has warned us that people with a brain injury often develop unusual eating habits. Sometimes, because of poor memory, they'll forget that they've already eaten and will eat two or three meals in a row; at other times, they may forget to eat altogether.

Daniel unloads the dishwasher without even being asked. He is so anxious to feel useful that he willingly helps now. I hold my breath each time he carries a stack of dishes across the room to the cupboard. It's a calculated risk, but one I'm prepared to take. What are a few broken dishes compared to his increased self-esteem?

Afterwards, when Daniel asks me to attach the muscle stimulator to his leg, I set him up on the couch in the family room. It's much easier to do this at home, instead of in his bed at the rehab centre. At least here he can watch TV instead of staring at a blank ceiling.

"I'm going out with the dog for a walk," I tell him. "Be back by the time you're done."

The leaves have started to change colours to cranberry, pumpkin, and mustard yellow. A few are swept by the light breeze into my path and crunch underfoot. The crackling sound reminds me of walking with the kids at the cottage in early frost past shallow puddles rimmed with ice. Too inviting to ignore: a small sneakered foot would tap at the edges, crack the glassy surface with textured whorls like an icy fingerprint. I walk briskly, pleased to be outside, to have a few moments of freedom. The dog trots along beside me.

That evening at dinner, when Daniel tries to sit in the seat at the foot of the table, Jonathan jockeys him aside. "Sit in your own spot."

"This is *my* place," says Daniel.

"No, it's mine. You're not in a wheelchair anymore."

Suddenly it feels as if I have two oversized kids. Out of practice living together, the boys continue to jostle each other. Daniel grabs his brother's hat and refuses to give it back. I'm starting to get annoyed.

Where is Joel when I need him? I pause and remember — he's playing squash tonight, a well-deserved break.

My sons' bickering brings to mind the voices of Al and Marilyn's little kids at their chalet last winter. You thought your house too quiet then, I remind myself. Still, I insist that Daniel return Jonathan's cap and encourage him to take his old seat beside me. Somehow we get through the meal without any further mishaps.

As we start to clear the table, I ask, "Do you guys want lasagne for dinner tomorrow night?"

"No, let's have pizza," says Jonathan.

Daniel nods enthusiastically, "Yes, pizza."

When I agree, Jonathan gives his brother an exuberant high five. "Daniel, it always takes two votes to convince her. I'm glad you're here."

After dinner, Daniel and I set up the chessboard in the kitchen and sit across from one another. He positions his right hand on the table, pressing first on his wrist and then on his joints, trying to straighten out his curling fingers. At night, before he goes to bed, we help him strap on a plastic hand brace that keeps his right fingers spread. It seems strange that my children are now all left-handed. Had Daniel been born a leftie like his brother and sister, he wouldn't have had to switch after his injury.

Maybe one day he'll regain more functional use of his right hand. He's working so hard at it. As he's relaxing or watching TV, he'll often exercise with therapy putty that feels a lot like Play-Doh. Somewhere in my files, I bet there's still a recipe for making Play-Doh: flour, water, salt, cream of tartar, and food colouring. I remember my kids would sit for hours at the kitchen table rolling out snake shapes, wrapping coils, pinching and squeezing out imaginary delicacies that they pretended to eat.

Daniel lines up his row of pawns confidently, and then fusses with the other chess pieces. When he misaligns the knights and bishops, I shift them around. That much I can do, along with guiding the basic moves. To get better training in strategy, he'll need to play with his father.

I like the way that Joel and I share responsibility for helping our son, and as in everything else we do, we tend to specialize. I focus on educational skills, games, and household tasks; Joel deals with the legal and insurance issues, and takes Daniel swimming three times a week.

Still, I'm concerned about how Daniel will spend his evenings now that he's living at home. At the rehab centre, there were always scheduled activities with the other patients under the guidance of a recreational therapist: organized games in the lounge or gym, snack preparation, or supervision for using the Internet program *Ability OnLine*, a chat room for students with disabilities. Neither Joel nor I want to become his personal recreational therapist. Jonathan is lobbying for a pool table and promises to play with Daniel every day if we buy them one. Alyssa, more practical, suggests we buy more Nintendo games that Daniel can play by himself.

Daniel would love to be constantly surrounded by his peers and is so upbeat when they come to visit. But he can't always count on them. His friend Jeff dropped by late Sunday morning. The sounds of laughter and ping-pong wafting from our basement reminded me of how things used to be, a bittersweet feeling. When another friend scheduled to come by at 2:00 p.m. didn't show, I'm not sure who was more disappointed, Daniel or I.

In our professional lives, my husband and I keep a schedule where time commitments are an integral part of successful performance. Even our social lives revolve around time — dinner with friends at 6:30 p.m., the play or concert starting at 8:00 p.m. We live our lives with one eye on the clock. Daniel's friends are different; Alyssa's too. More fluid, more spontaneous. "I'll be there at 7," can mean they show at 8. But Daniel has become a stickler for time.

On Sunday he was invited to a gathering at someone's house and was expecting to be picked up at 8:30 p.m. He checked his watch every five minutes. At 9:15 p.m. he asked anxiously, "Where are they?"

Had they forgotten him? Changed their minds? Run into a problem? I wondered.

At 9:20 p.m. the doorbell finally rang, and Daniel hurried to answer it. Teddy greeted him with a wrap-around hug. Jared and Jaimie were standing there too, smiling, oblivious to the worry they'd caused. Greetings, a handshake, then a fast goodbye.

That night, I lay awake with my bedside lamp on, reading and waiting. Waiting for the sound of the front door to open. Precisely at 1:00 a.m., the pre-arranged time, I heard a click of the lock, then my son's voice, "It was great. See you."

I listened to the clump of his uneven footsteps as he limped up the stairs, past my doorway, and down the hall to his room. When I heard his door close, I took a deep breath and turned out the light.

CHAPTER THIRTY-SEVEN

One Saturday morning in late October, I'm jarred awake by the buzz of the intercom that connects our bedroom to Daniel's. Something is wrong, I fear, as I scurry down the hall to his room. I look around anxiously. It's a peaceful scene. Daniel is reclining in bed with a book in his hand. It's a thin paperback with a picture of the movie star of *The Karate Kid* on the cover.

"What's this?" asks Daniel.

"The book you were reading."

"But I stopped," he says, noting the bookmark midway through.

"Yes, you couldn't remember what was happening."

Daniel started reading this book in August. Joel and I are always reading something at the cottage, and Daniel wanted to, also. So I gave him this book. I thought he could handle it because it's written at a grade four or five level, the same reading level as he was working on in class. I learned that Daniel could read most of the words correctly, but he struggled to understand the main idea and to recall the details of the story. So I worked with him, making summary notes of each chapter that we reviewed before he read the next. This system worked well for a while. However, in September, when his classes resumed at Hugh Mac, Daniel complained to his speech pathologist that reading felt too much like homework. She suggested that we discontinue the practice of note taking, and that he just read on his own for pleasure.

He tried. Yet, shortly afterwards, I noticed that he gave up reading at home altogether. I tried not to get discouraged.

Now with the book in his hand, Daniel says, "Tell me what it's about."

I take the book from him, extract my notes for chapters one to five, and recount the highlights. He smiles as the memory of some of the details comes back to him.

"I like this story. What happened next?"

"I don't know. I didn't read that part. Daniel, you have to have notes or you'll forget what you're reading."

"Will I ever get better?"

"Yes," I say hopefully, thinking of his teacher's comments: Daniel is making slow but steady progress.

"Then I'll wait to get better." He leans towards his night table to replace the book, then hesitates. "No. I'd better read now, so I'll make it better. Will you help?"

His response delights me. I'm not surprised that he wants to start immediately. His teacher and therapists are all impressed by my son's positive attitude and determination.

We start with chapter six. He can't read quickly enough to skim the material himself, so I read aloud chunks of information to him, pausing so we can paraphrase it and make notes. I can see that he's tiring, yet he wants to go on.

I wrestle the book from him. "We'll do more later," I promise. "Let's eat breakfast."

When Daniel started at Hugh Mac last winter, his first academic challenge was learning to focus and maintain his attention. He was distracted by the other students in the classroom, although there were only three of them. With a teacher's aide at his side for guidance, he began practising basic addition and subtraction facts — a far cry from the calculus course that was giving him grief in the semester before his injury. Now he's worked his way up to multiplication and division examples. When I observed him in class last week, I asked his teacher what the purpose was. Why not just give him a calculator and teach him to use that? Wouldn't it be simpler? She explained that computation practice is meant to develop organization and sequencing skills, with the expectation that these skills will transfer to other areas.

Reading, writing, math — there are so many foundation skills to rebuild.

I've been trying to get a laptop computer from the Writing Aids clinic for Daniel to use while he's still at the rehab centre. His occupational therapist started the process months ago, knowing it would be helpful to have his teacher or her assistant experiment with the various software programs, evaluating their effectiveness before we made any decision about what to buy. Even with a computer, Daniel will need to brainstorm his ideas with someone before writing a first draft, and he'll need help with the editing process. I've witnessed this firsthand when working with him at home on my computer. He has such difficulty expressing his ideas coherently in writing — a form of aphasia — and often can't correct words that are identified as misspelled even when alternatives are given.

Daniel wants to continue his studies and still expects to complete the one high school credit he needs to graduate. But I worry about finding him an appropriate educational placement when he leaves the rehab centre in December. There are no specialized programs anywhere around for students with brain injury. His teacher and I have started exploring the possibilities with a representative from the school board: an orthopaedic program, a learning disabilities class, or a school for slow learners. I immediately reject the latter. Not only is the class size too large — fifteen to twenty students with no teacher's assistant — it would be devastating for Daniel's self-esteem.

His teacher says that Daniel responds best with structure and cueing before tackling an activity independently, so the learning disabilities class might work. It has the right philosophy. Then we learn that the class is in a "tough school." The implication is obvious. With his physical handicaps, Daniel might have a difficult time fitting in with the other students. No way do I want him to be bullied or ridiculed. I feel like a protective lioness about to roar as she senses a threat to her cub.

We're trying to consider all his needs: physical, cognitive, social, and emotional. A challenging prospect. We're soon left with just one option — the orthopaedic class. But Daniel's physical deficits are the least defining of his problems right now. It feels as if we're trying to fit a square peg into a round hole. That's what brain injury is like. In our discussions, Joel has been highly sceptical of the school board's ability to meet Daniel's needs. It seems he's right.

One afternoon, I take Daniel to Discoverability, a career-counselling centre for the physically disabled, to explore other options. I share his teacher's notes with the counsellor and seek her advice. She focusses on the starred comment — needs one-to-one support for best results — but doesn't notice his current academic functioning level. When I discreetly circle it for her, Daniel detects my actions and asks me for the results. His face looks pained when I answer.

"Grade five?" he repeats. "All my friends are in university now. That's where I should be."

I try to keep my voice composed. "Look how far you've come, and you're still making progress."

Daniel is only somewhat mollified. He barely pays attention when the counsellor confirms Joel's belief that a private remedial education centre would be best for this next phase of our son's education.

Then she says, "It's too soon to do career planning right now. Let's wait and see how you do in school. We can meet again next September."

When Daniel leaves the room to go to the washroom, I ask her whether he could be considered for the Teen Independence Program this coming summer. This monthlong, live-in course is geared to helping students with a physical disability make the transition from high school to college or university. It targets independent living skills and includes opportunities for banking, budgeting, shopping, cooking, and learning to live with peers. Last August when I observed the program in a downtown university residence, Joel and I naïvely hoped that Daniel would progress so much that he wouldn't need it. It's terribly painful to hear the counsellor say that at this stage Daniel wouldn't even be eligible. Still, she leaves me with a window of possibility.

"We don't know how much progress he'll make from now to May when interviews take place. Let's wait and see."

Wait and see. I can't lasso the hope. It slips from my grasp as, once again, I realize we have to readjust our plans and our dreams. Daniel is making tiny steps, baby steps of progress. And the distance he wants to travel is so great.

TENTH NEWSLETTER

November 13, 1994
Dear Family and Friends,

I've had a lot of trouble writing this newsletter. The anecdotes I usually include do not seem adequate to paint an accurate picture of Daniel. Now that he's living at home with us and is becoming more a part of the community, we have a sense of conflicting messages. The young man looks like a miracle to those of you who have watched or followed what he's been through these past fourteen months. But he looks like a handicapped person to the general public who see him for the first time. It's hard for them to ignore the visible differences and to be aware of the invisible effects of head injury.

Yet this lack of awareness affects you as well. We are constantly being told how great Daniel looks. While it's true, don't be fooled into thinking that because he looks great and continues to improve that everything is fine. Yes, it's a miracle that he's walking, talking, and interacting so well. But we want more — so much more.

Joel and I talk non-stop. Every day, we rehash what Daniel said and did, looking for signs that suggest continued improvement. When we see him on a daily basis, it's hard to be aware of these gains. It's like watching a young child grow: all of a sudden, you realize that his or her clothes don't fit. What we keep wanting are guarantees that the flashes of insight we see are signals of potential that will yet be realized. Whenever Alyssa comes into Toronto, about every second or third weekend, she notices differences that are not always obvious to us.

Physically, Daniel continues to make good progress. He has given up his wheelchair and now walks with a cane. Yet, when he's manoeuvring his way around the kitchen, setting the table, or carrying food, he manages to walk steadily without any aid at all. Although his right hand and arm are slowly improving, his left hand has become the dominant one. It's now strong enough to deal with all those hard-to-open jars that I can't handle. He still talks out of the left side of his mouth, but his smile is once again a full smile.

His memory for functional tasks has improved tremendously — he can go through his daily routines independently, as well as remind us to feed the dog or buy his favourite cereal.

So what do we worry about? It's often difficult to assess how much he's processing from an ordinary conversation. Has he understood all the words and concepts? Will he focus just on the concrete, or can he pick up some of the nuances and inferences? When more than one person is speaking, can he follow as the conversation jumps back and forth with sentences often left incomplete or interrupted? We're also concerned about his academic skills. They are slow to return.

Daniel was discharged as an in-patient at Hugh Mac on October 7 and has been living at home full-time since then. He'll continue to receive therapy there as an outpatient until mid-December. The first week Daniel was home we were euphoric. I didn't even mind when Daniel and Jonathan started to argue over seats at the table and snatched each other's napkins. Normal sibling fighting — what a treat! Then the reality hit. Daniel has become more assertive and is striving for independence. We're still not comfortable leaving him for an extended period unsupervised; we're trying to maintain a balance between safety and letting go.

He's been involved in our discussions about future schooling and rehabilitation. Starting in January, he'll be receiving two hours of daily tutoring at a private learning centre. Three or four times a week he'll head out to a rehab centre for physio and occupational therapy. We must still find the time to schedule his speech and language therapy and music therapy. We'll definitely need a driver if I'm to continue working.

For all our concerns and worries, what seems most obvious to us are not Daniel's disabilities, but his zest for life, his re-emerging personality, and his sense of humour. His motivation and incredible determination will keep the progress flowing. He is planning to try downhill skiing again this winter with a group called Adult Disabled Downhill Skiing and is already talking about water-skiing next summer. He wants to get a head start on the season by skiing with a wetsuit in May or June.

With so many of his friends out of town at university, our long distance bills are high as he tries to keep in touch with them.

Last week, Jonathan was saddened upon seeing a picture of his brother in a friend's album. The picture was from two summers ago, before Daniel's injury. When Daniel heard the story, he patted Jonathan on his shoulder and reassured him, "Don't worry, I'm coming back!"

Love,
Lainie

CHAPTER THIRTY-EIGHT

The sun is stingy with its rays at this time of year, late November. It shines through the bare trees, crafting thin shadows. It emits little warmth. I shiver, even indoors. I'm filled with trepidation, anticipating our meeting at the rehab centre to get the results of Daniel's neuropsychological assessment. It feels almost like a trial to me, waiting to have a verdict delivered. I'm hoping that the results will confirm the prediction the neurosurgeon made the night of Daniel's operation, "Your son will have a good life," she had said.

But what does that mean? Joel and I have already adjusted our sights from expecting Daniel to go to university, to hoping he'll complete his last credit for high school. And I'm not sure if even that goal is feasible. Yet Daniel hasn't changed his mind. University was something he took for granted. And he expected to leave town to do it. He still assumes that when he graduates from high school, he'll move on. Move away from home like his sister and many of his friends have. Move on with his life.

I wish he could. Daniel's lack of insight is both a blessing and a concern. He really wants to be able to pick up his life the way it was. But he can't go back.

What does the future hold for him? We still dream that somehow he'll have an independent life, a meaningful vocation, a lasting relationship. That's what we dream of for all our children. But there are no guarantees.

Alyssa, whose course was so steady with her desire to follow her father into accountancy, now talks of other options. She doesn't want to commit to any more studies when she completes her senior year in the business program. Perhaps when she graduates, she'll work — she doesn't know at what — and then travel. She'll see, she says.

Jonathan's goals are much more immediate — to make the competitive hockey team and to try out for basketball in the spring. He's more concerned about when he'll grow facial hair and need to shave than he is about higher education or his vocation. We're not too worried. Jonathan has plenty of time to make those decisions.

I'm in a lounge chair waiting outside the neuropsychologist's office when Joel arrives for our meeting at 4:00 p.m. He looks composed, not like me. I've been crossing one leg, then the other, trying to get comfortable. When he sits beside me, I squeeze his hand.

"Your hand is freezing," he says. He takes my fingers in his and rubs them gently.

Mary opens her office door, greets us, and ushers us in. She takes a seat behind her desk with her back to the window; we settle across from her — similar to the position we had a year ago when we were discussing Daniel's prognosis with his neurosurgeon in her office. It seems a lifetime ago.

The waning sunlight glints through the window, accenting the waves in Mary's dark hair. Her head bobs as she looks from one of us to the other, then back to Daniel's file. She begins talking in a fluid tone, methodically describing the test results and the suggested implications.

My hands are tucked into the pockets of my jacket draped over my shoulders. I'm not taking notes today. We'll get a written copy of her report. My fingers locate something metallic in the righthand pocket — a paper clip — and rub it like an amulet.

Although Joel and I are aware of most of Daniel's deficits, particularly in the language area, I'm not prepared to hear just how widespread the damage is and how devastating the repercussions associated with it. Mary explains that Daniel needs all information presented to him in a highly structured format. During testing, the examiner uses signals and repetition to present the material. Without these modifications, Daniel would have significant difficulty with information processing and problem solving. His injury has affected his visual spatial skills too; skills that I assumed would be a strength for him. The only areas still relatively intact are his social relationships and appropriate behaviour.

Thank heavens for small mercies. These skills may be the ones he will need most to lead a functional life. A few weeks ago, I overheard Daniel on the phone with Alyssa, making plans to visit her in London. He had already invited his friends to her apartment for a party to celebrate his birthday. He'll take the train, he said, not at all concerned about travelling alone. I can picture how we marked the occasion of his eighteenth birthday — propping him up in a seated position in his hospital bed. This year's celebration will be immeasurably better.

Joel is not nearly as upset by the meeting as I am. He maintains a healthy scepticism when it comes to hearing results from experts.

"Test results are just a snapshot in time," he says.

I know that. I often use this phrase myself in feedback meetings with parents. My days are spent assessing students, then using those results as one source of data to help the school team make decisions about educational programming and placement. At times now, I find myself becoming more cautious at work, couching my conclusions, and seeking more confirmation from the family as to how they view their son or daughter.

"The experts have been wrong before," Joel reminds me. "The Evoked Potential Tests and CAT scans suggested that Daniel wouldn't ever reach the level he's at now. Remember that doctor who predicted that Daniel wouldn't even know his own name or who we are?"

My stomach recoils at the memory. No one can tell us how much of our son's progress can be attributed to spontaneous recovery and how much to his intensive rehabilitation training — training of which we're such an integral part. No one can measure the value of the support of his friends or the effect of his own determination. And no one can tell us just how far Daniel will go. Joel's attitude is still "shoot for the stars." It's his undiminished hope that keeps him going. In contrast, my constant reality check mires me in recurring sorrow.

Our society doesn't condone public grieving, and it is especially hard to grieve openly for someone who is still alive. I'm supposed to count my blessings, to be thankful for all the good in my life. And there are many wonderful things to count. But that doesn't remove my pain. It cloaks it, hides it, but grief demands its turn to be heard, like an angry little child stamping her foot if no one pays her enough attention.

I was standing in front of a display of grapes in the supermarket one afternoon, when my tears came unbidden, tiny globes of salted water streaming from my eyes. I stood frozen in place. Looked around in a panic. There was nowhere to hide. Would some stranger approach me? Would the P.A. system announce, "Lady having breakdown in aisle one? Please bring a mop."

Go away, grief! I didn't invite you. I don't want you now.

So I fill my life with busyness, with doing, hoping I won't have to visit the pain that grief brings. Sometimes I complain of Daniel hammering away at issues that bother him. It seems I do the same, only I call it research and analysis. I read everything I can about outpatient rehab and educational facilities. And I've started collecting stories. Friends keep giving me the names of people they've heard about — a neighbour, a cousin's friend, a colleague — that have experienced brain injury in their families. I call these strangers — I, who always hated to make phone calls to solicit donations for the charitable organizations I volunteered for. I hate cold calls.

The people on the other end of the phone are so willing to talk to me. I seek road markings, shortcuts to pursue, and pitfalls to avoid. There is no map to follow. With the brain being the most complex organ in our body, it's not surprising that the constellation of deficits is unique for each individual who sustains a brain injury. The family members can't give me specific advice to help Daniel; instead they share stories of their own loved one.

Yet despite their openness, I can't ask these strangers the one question I'd really like answered: How long does it take for acceptance to come?

Joel and I believe that we're coping well with our problems. Friends admire our outward strength and sense of purpose. However, in some ways it appears that we're just working hard to deny the reality: the impact of this horrible tragedy in our lives. Are we supposed to handle this differently? Should we cry more? Get angry? Would that help?

We have started seeing a therapist together, one who's associated with the rehab centre. In our bi-weekly visits, we can barely scratch the surface of all that's bothering us. Eva tells us that the second year following a trauma such as Daniel's is in some ways more difficult than the first. After the initial shock of the experience comes the realization that there is no magic cure for brain injury.

I thought that the counselling sessions would serve primarily as an educational process to help us set realistic goals for Daniel. However, for me, they've become the time to express my concerns and to grieve openly. Sometimes when my fears are exposed, the chasm created seems wide enough to swallow me up. It's scary to face.

And there's still John's preliminary hearing to get through.

CHAPTER THIRTY-NINE

"The courthouse is right across from the emerald palace," the prosecutor's secretary tells me. "You can't miss it."

As I drive north on Yonge Street in early December, I look for it — a modern office building of concrete and glass with green tinted windows that glint in the sun. The secretary is right. You can't miss its glow or the tall clock tower that beckons like a beacon. Across the street, the courthouse looks drab by comparison, like a poor relative dressed in shabby brown. The tiered brick building sprawls behind a muddied lawn patched with snow. I wind down the driveway and park my car.

Do I really want to do this? I ask myself. John has been formally charged with the offence of dangerous driving causing bodily harm.

The prosecutor invited us to attend the preliminary hearing, where the Crown will try to establish that there's enough evidence to take this case to trial. We're not obligated to be present. Joel claimed he had a conflicting meeting that couldn't be changed. I could have begged off too, or at least arranged for someone to come with me. Ellen would have come gladly if only I had asked her. But I'm tired of being on the receiving end with all my friends, especially Ellen. She's put herself out so much already.

So I'm here alone, somehow needing to hear the case first-hand, to find out what really happened that fateful summer day. I brace myself before walking past the rows of pine trees that guard the steps of the building. It feels like I'm walking a gauntlet. Once inside, I'm not sure where to go. An oak-railed staircase leads upstairs and down.

"Where is court two?" I ask a security guard, and then proceed in the pointed direction.

It's awkward standing by myself in the lobby, waiting for the proceedings to begin. Even worse, when John walks over to me with Daniel's friend, Jaimie. What did I expect? That Jaimie and the other guys would abandon John? Blame him for causing Daniel's injuries?

Joel has not forgiven John for driving so recklessly. At first, Daniel was unaware of his friend's actions and welcomed John's visits. Yet, about eight months post-injury, when Daniel regained his voice and greater awareness, he told John to stop visiting.

"You did this to me!" he accused his friend.

For the next several months, Daniel held on to those feelings of anger and reproach. Then, with the help of a therapist, he developed greater understanding of his own culpability for not wearing his seatbelt, for not asking his friend to drive slower. Eventually, he released John from blame. But Daniel decided that he didn't want to renew their friendship, "We can be friendly, but not friends."

Today, John and Jaimie greet me warmly. They've traded their jeans for dark pants and their T-shirts for dress shirts. John wears a tie. We chat about the unseasonably cold weather, the early snow, and the prospect it brings for a good season of skiing.

Chitter chatter, this doesn't matter, I recite silently like some nursery rhyme.

Four adults approach. I recognize one woman from my synagogue. John introduces me to the others: his divorced parents and his lawyer. The woman with the familiar face turns out to be his father's fiancée. I shake their hands and wish them well.

I'm glad that Joel isn't here today. He couldn't bring himself to do this — to wish them well. Yet, when the lawyer from the prosecutor's office asked whether we'd like to see a two-year jail sentence imposed if John were convicted, we both said no. We're not looking to make John or his family suffer needlessly. Revenge won't change anything.

The lawyer tried to plead her case, "You would deter other drivers from making the same mistake."

But I don't believe a jail term for John would have any impact at all on other drivers. Young men are often impulsive. Sometimes they drive recklessly and aggressively despite all our societal and parental warnings. Alyssa reminds us how easily it could have been her brother behind the wheel of a car doing the same thing.

The court is called into session. John's mother invites me to sit with them, but I can't do that. I watch John and his entourage proceed to the front of the room. They sit together in a solid line. I slip into a seat midway up the aisle.

Why am I here? The pending outcome has no direct impact on us. Nor can it change the outcome for Daniel. Sometimes I wish it were that simple. That some judge could pound her gavel and deliver a verdict giving Daniel a second chance. It doesn't seem fair. My older son has learned his lesson. Must he pay for his mistake for the rest of his life? Must we? Are we destined to a lifetime devoted to rehabilitating him?

Some friends suggest we get on with our own lives. That message sounds so harsh to me. Can't they understand that our lives are so intricately tied up to Daniel's right now that we can't imagine living any other way?

The director of the adolescent unit of the rehab centre compares living with a child with a severe brain injury to running a long distance marathon. He's seen many parents plunge full steam ahead and then burn out quickly.

"Pace yourself," he advises. "Take time to refuel. You're in it for the long run."

We're trying. Yet, we've chosen to ignore the social worker's suggestion to hire a case manager to coordinate the services that Daniel will need when he is discharged from the centre.

"A case manager can give you emotional distance," Bob says. "Ease your load."

But Joel and I don't want to have information filtered to us through someone else. We want to communicate directly with the therapists, lawyers, and insurance agents, to have some sense of control over the process. I've spoken to some other parents at the brain injury association who feel the same way. They, too, have done what we're planning — do it themselves.

I glance around the wood-panelled courtroom. It's almost empty. A couple in their late fifties. A policeman in uniform. Was he the one at the accident scene, the one who called Alyssa with the news?

Two men walk by me. One is young; the other one, middle-aged, carries a briefcase like John's lawyer. The lawyers here are in suits. Only the judge, sitting at the front of the room, bears the solemn weight of black-robed tradition over his shoulders.

The first witness is called to the stand. With his trim grey hair and dark blue blazer, he has the stolid demeanour of an upright citizen. The lawyer for the prosecution asks him to testify about the events that he recalls leading up to the car crash on the afternoon of August 29.

"I was driving at my normal speed. With my wife in the car, I never go faster than the posted speed limit." He tugs on his shirt collar as if it had suddenly tightened. His face reddens a little. "Well, sometimes a little faster, maybe, but not that day. The radio was on and we were talking. I didn't hear the other car at first. Then there it was in my rear-view mirror — a small black car bearing down on us. I couldn't tell the make, although afterwards I was told it was a Volkswagen Golf. It was really speeding. 'Where does he think he's going?' I asked my wife. You see, I was in the left lane, but the lanes merge just ahead. The car pulled up on my right just as the right lane ends. The driver couldn't pull back. He was going too fast. He hit the shoulder and then everything happened so quickly."

An accident is an event without apparent cause. This was no accident!

He pauses and takes a sip of water. "Did it pass ahead of me or behind me, you ask? Behind me, I think. Yes, definitely, behind me."

The prosecutor stands and asks another question.

The witness gulps like a fish out of water.

"I can't say for certain what happened next."

My heart is speeding up like that black car, just from listening to the testimony. I peer at John's parents, at the back of their heads that remain statue-like facing the front. Are they wondering why their son drove so irresponsibly? What was John thinking?

When the prosecutor releases the witness, the man squares his shoulders, nods to the judge, and rejoins his wife.

The second witness is called up. He states his name and address quickly — Ozzie something — I don't quite catch it. He's a young man of Asian background, probably in his mid-twenties. Hard to tell. His face is smooth and round, but his voice has an excited quality to it. He answers questions about speed, distance, and other facts like a racehorse anxious to leave the gate, restrained by the reins. Now he's galloping, filling in the gaps in the story.

"All of a sudden, there was gravel spraying and this car careened across the road, ahead of me maybe two hundred yards. It flipped, spinning and twirling. Two people were thrown. A scary sight. I stopped my car and rushed out. The driver was moaning; the passenger silent, but bleeding a lot. I checked the car to see if there was anyone else in it. Then I dashed back to my car. I had no cellphone so I drove to the next turnoff, pulled into someone's driveway to call the police. The owner of the house gave me a quilt to cover the passenger. I figured he'd be in shock."

So that's where the quilt came from. The white quilt with patterned swirls darkened by blood — my son's blood. Tagged as Daniel's property, we had picked it up from the first hospital the ambulance had taken him to. Not knowing what else to do, I washed it and tucked it away on a shelf in my linen closet, expecting to return it some day. But the police couldn't tell me where it came from.

Ozzie is reaching the finish line and my stomach is about to betray me. I rush out of the courtroom to a toilet stall. Along with the diarrhoea, I feel nauseous and faint as well. I lower my head below my knees and wait for the vertigo to pass.

That stupid kid! This didn't have to happen.

When I finally make my way to a sink, I see John's future stepmother standing nearby, wiping her hands. She looks at me solicitously and asks if I'm all right. I splash cold water onto my whitened face and don't answer. She waits anxiously, looking as if she's about to reach out and touch me. Recoiling, I cringe and say, "I'm okay," then I hurry out of the courthouse.

The cold air immediately stings my lungs. Guzzling in deep breaths, I can't seem to get enough of it. I don't bother to button my jacket, just wrap it tightly closed. Now I'm beside my car. My hand is shaking and the key won't fit into the door lock. I fumble around until finally I'm seated in the front seat with the ignition on. Blasts of cold air attack me through the heating vents. The windows fog up. As I wait for them to clear, I'm startled to hear a knock on my side window. I rub a spot and peer through. Jaimie is there, shivering with his unfastened jacket, his face a warm smile. I open the window and before he can say anything, I assure him that I'm fine. Liar.

"I'll let you know how things go," says Jaimie. "And tell Daniel I'll be there tomorrow. I'm going to spend today with John."

Some things in life are reasonably predictable. Others are not. Weeks after John's preliminary hearing, we learn the outcome from Jaimie. Although there's enough evidence to take this case to trial, the matter has been settled. Apparently John has pleaded guilty to a lesser charge; Jaimie wasn't specific. And the judge followed most of our recommendations for sentencing. John won't have to serve a jail term. He'll perform three hundred hours of community service and his driver's license will be suspended for three years. We had asked for five.

I don't know whether John ever completed the sentence. A year or so later, we heard that he was moving to the United States with his father and stepmother. When he returned to Toronto once for a visit, he and Daniel met at a party and treated each other, not as long-lost friends, but as someone each dimly recalled.

That day in the courthouse, I couldn't imagine the trip I would take nearly five years later. I was on a leave of absence from my job because I was feeling almost burned out from all the responsibilities I shouldered. Finally with some time to devote to myself, I started to explore my own needs. I took long reflective walks, enrolled in a writing course, and began to dream of snow-capped mountains.

Then one day, there I was, with a group of strangers flying halfway around the world to the mountains of Nepal. In a tiny plane that dipped through fluffy clouds I watched the peaks unzip, revealing a secret opening. Hillsides were scalloped stepping stones, a puzzle of green and brown, and a silver line far below looked scratched by a giant's stick.

Day followed day through lush forests of tall pines and giant rhododendrons, then the scenery changed to dried scruffy hills. I trod up and down steep paths of dirt and stone, curling roots, browning pine needles, gauging my tread over jagged rocks. My guide walked in flip-flops, his step so sure, his breath so even, while mine was laboured and ragged. I passed houses of stone, plastered white and painted with windows of blue or earthy orange. In the courtyards, round trays of millet and racks of pale corncobs dried in the sun, beside a mangy dog curled asleep in the dirt. Children ran out of the houses, their palms joined across their chests. *"Namaste,"* they called out in greeting, delighting in my response. In the distant foreground were the snow-capped tips of the Himalayas, coyly beckoning behind a veil of clouds.

I'd lie in my tent at night in a field and would drift to sleep to the sounds of drumming and chanting of the villagers nearby. One day, when I awakened, I discovered that the ground and my tent were rimed with frost. As I sipped a cup of steaming tea, I gazed at the sun slowly rising behind the distant hills. A weak yellow, not yet golden bright, glistened on the frozen grass and lit up the horizon, vanishing the grey skies. I knew then how much I was looking forward to seeing my family again. I missed them: Joel, Alyssa, Jonathan, my mother, and Daniel — Daniel, as he is now, not as he used to be. My steps were steadier when I headed off.

Epilogue

How does this story end? I wanted to be able to say that we lived happily ever after like the characters in fairy tales I used to favour as a child. For a long time, I was reluctant to even begin writing this book as I kept waiting for that fantasy ending. Finally, I realized that there could be no ending at all, no definitive resolution to this event, just a re-telling of the journey itself.

My original purpose in writing this book was to record Daniel's story, to give him a sense of what happened to him in the first year following his injury. I had hoped to fill in the gaps in his memory so he could appreciate just how far he'd come. However, as I started to write, I realized that the journey was really my own. As a wife, mother, and daughter, it became clear to me that the story was about my whole family, for what happened to Daniel affected us all.

I remember, as if it were yesterday, that first night following surgery when we watched my son's chest rise and fall in rhythmic breathing, thankful he was alive. We couldn't imagine then how we would cope with this trauma, yet somehow we did. Helped by the love and support of family and friends, we waited and watched, hoped and prayed. To survive, we picked up the pieces and plunged ahead, often blindly feeling our way, not knowing what forks in the road awaited. Although we have tried to stay focussed in the moment and live one day at a time, that's still a tall order for us. Some days are better than others — the ones when we remind ourselves to appreciate what we have. But we can't stop scanning that road ahead, anticipating what might happen next.

Three years after Daniel's injury, we sat in a large auditorium with other parents of the 1996 York Mills high school graduating class. Daniel was dressed in a suit that evening — a handsome double-breasted green silk suit that his uncle Yaron had given him. Yet when I looked at my son, I pictured him wearing his favourite T-shirt emblazoned across the back with a saying that epitomizes his attitude to life, "It's not how good you are, it's how bad you want it."

When Daniel was finally discharged from the rehab centre after his eleven-month stay, we took a family holiday in Mexico. We had reserved a wheelchair for him to use in the airport, but he insisted on walking everywhere. Daniel didn't remember ever travelling in an airplane before (retrograde amnesia can do that), so everything was a new experience for him. He was like a sponge, absorbing all the sights and sounds around him trying to make up for lost time.

Once we were settled at the hotel, Daniel warned me that he

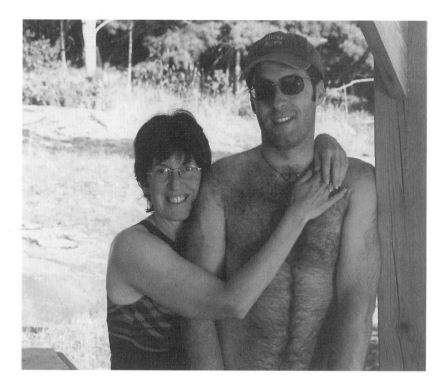

Lainie and Daniel at the cottage, summer 2002

might not have much time to spend with us, as he intended to socialize. And mingle he did! When Joel and I were heading to bed at night, our three children were gearing up for the disco. Daniel had no qualms about asking girls to dance, and with his cane left by his chair, he was in the thick of things. What he enjoyed most though was being in the ocean with Alyssa and Jonathan, for with a lifejacket on he, too, had the freedom to ride the waves.

The next spring, Daniel announced he would try water-skiing.

His first few attempts were unsuccessful, and although he was disappointed, he wasn't prepared to give up. He increased his daily program of exercises to further strengthen his right arm and leg and improve his balance. At the cottage, he tried "tubing" — being pulled behind the boat while lying on an inflated tube — but he was determined to ski again.

One summer weekend, our friend, David, provided his ski boat with all the necessary accessories: the skis, a boom and a shortened rope, his driving experience, and incredible patience. Another friend, Andrew, a trained water-ski instructor, came up to our cottage for the weekend to provide special hands-on instruction and in-the-water support. Joel was in the boat helping, Alyssa worked the video camera, and I sat on the dock being nervous. At first, all Daniel could do was crouch and hold onto the boom before falling. After a few attempts, fatigue set in. Finally, many trials later, he made it up to a standing position. His smile was worth all the effort and symbolized an important milestone. His graduation ceremony heralded another.

The graduates were announced with their current university programs, scholarship standings, and many awards. My son had none of these. Yet when Daniel limped across that stage and stretched out his left hand to receive his diploma, there were many wet eyes around. We stood with all the others in the audience, proudly applauding his determination and drive. We didn't know then that in a few months time, Daniel would regain his coveted driver's license, and that Joel and I would spend almost one hundred hours in the car practising with him to help him achieve it.

Whenever Daniel's set a goal for himself, we've been there to help.

In one therapist's office, a plaque over the doorway reads, "Those who say it cannot be done, should not interrupt those who are doing it." We've tried to follow that motto. However, sometimes even we underestimate him.

In the winter of 1998, we went skiing at Silver Star in the Okanagan Valley in British Columbia. Jonathan and a friend spent each day racing down the expert hills; Daniel, Joel, and I worked our way down the intermediate runs. While Daniel was receiving individual instruction one morning, my husband and I headed over to the north side of the mountain to take a more challenging route. When we hit a patch of moguls, I said, "It's a good thing we didn't take Daniel here. This would be too hard for him."

Just up ahead, we suddenly noticed his black helmet bobbing between the mounds of snow. Slowly, carefully, he was mastering it too.

Not everything has been as success- ful as that ski run, and it's been diffi- cult for us to let go and watch him fail. As much as we'd like to smooth the way for him, we don't have that control. We can't protect him or

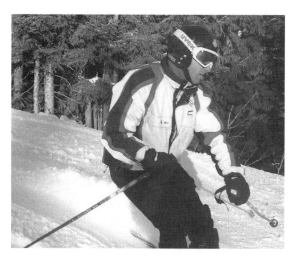

Daniel once again on the slopes

prevent the inevitable failures, disappointments, or setbacks.

Nor can I prevent the moments of grief that sometimes wash over me like a powerful wave. Even Daniel's triumphs, so hard earned, at times feel bittersweet. It's hard not to feel regret for what could have been, should have been. I recognize that these feelings soon ebb and like Daniel, I press forward.

My mother was diagnosed with cancer in the fall of 2001. She didn't survive to see this book in print, but she lived the story with us and left an indelible mark. When Ellen and I get together to walk or play golf, we often talk about our families. I'd like to believe my mother is somewhere listening and nodding her head.

Daniel is back in Toronto after two years at the Rusk Institute Brain Injury Day Treatment Program in New York. The Rusk program was successful in raising his awareness that a brain injury cannot be cured no matter how hard he tries. This painful message was tempered with training to apply compensatory strategies to reduce the impact of his deficits. Daniel has learned to carry around a notebook to aid in memory recall and to verify what people are saying to him to improve his understanding. More importantly, my son's inner qualities were highlighted — his determination, courage, and optimism; his sense of humour and zest for life. With an improved sense of acceptance of himself, Daniel does what he can to get the most out of life. He's currently living in his own apartment in a supported setting and recognizes that to live independently, he must count on others for support.

My youngest child, Jonathan, shares many of the same struggles

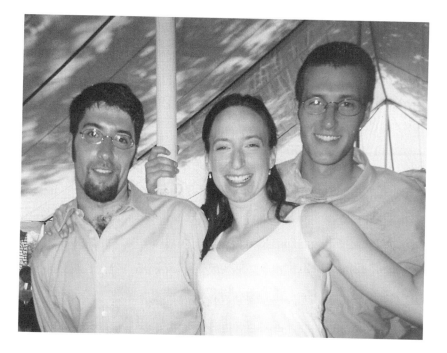

Daniel, Alyssa, and Jonathan at Alyssa's wedding, July 1999

for identity and purpose as Daniel. Jonathan realizes that he's not meant to be his brother's clone as he thought when he was young, nor must he feel guilty for enjoying the activities and everyday pleasures that often elude his older brother. He's trying to carve out a niche for himself, to get on with his own life. In the middle of his second semester at university, Jonathan decided to forgo his studies. He moved back home and seemed to flounder for a while, trying to build a business and working at odd jobs. Now he's back at college because he wants to be there. He shows an interest in business and a bent for creative writing. Who knows where his determination will take him?

My daughter, Alyssa, has not had a direct path, either. After graduating from university, she took some time off to focus on getting herself well and in her journey back to health, she decided to become a yoga teacher. Following eight months of travel through Europe, the Middle East, and India, she set up yoga classes in our basement, specializing in helping others who had chronic pain. In the summer of 1999, we were delighted to celebrate her marriage to a young man she met in her third year of university — the year of her brother's injury. After a brief stint as a manager for a large health resort in the U.S., Alyssa is now integrating her skills as the proud owner of her own yoga studio and healing therapies centre in Toronto. She and her husband, Scott, are expecting their first child.

I guess I could call this a happy ending. My family and my marriage are intact, something that no one predicted nine years ago. My children keep connected with each other through e-mail, phone calls, and visits to the cottage. And at the holidays, we again stand in front of the fireplace and whoever is in town joins the family photo.

Each summer when the anniversary date of August 29 approaches, I no longer anticipate it with dread, as I did the first year following Daniel's injury. We have turned it into a special occasion. We call it a celebration of life.

Four years ago, a few months after our dog Echo died, Joel and I went to choose a new puppy. Eight balls of flying fur came tumbling from the crate and skittered across the breeder's kitchen floor. Three hid beneath the raised wood stove. One bumped into a chair. We watched and waited, kneeling patiently. One puppy approached and climbed into my arms. Her body felt cuddly and warm. Joel held her

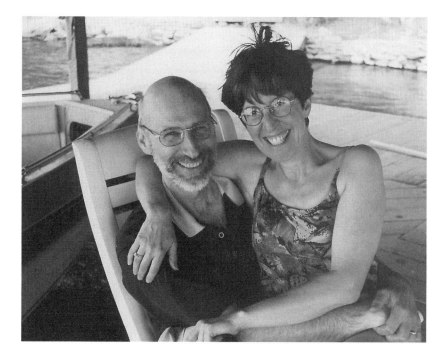

Lainie and Joel at the cottage, summer 1998

too and she licked his chin. When he placed her gently back on the floor, her shiny eyes and wagging tail confirmed her choice.

Whenever Joel and I go walking together in the woods near our cottage, we take Jazz, our golden retriever. We're aware of the change of seasons once again: the dense foliage of summer filtering the sun's hot rays, the crispness of autumn's leaves, the heavy tramping through paths hidden by winter's snow, and the freshness and promise of new buds in spring. Through it all, Jazz's ears flop up and down as she gambols ahead, stopping every now and again to make sure we're following.